Making Sense of the EEG

This book aims to educate the reader on the cellular and neurophysical aspects of electroencephalography (EEG), alongside its technical and engineering principles. Providing a background on normal EEG, this book covers the clinical applications of EEG in epilepsies and other brain disorders to provide the reader with the necessary knowledge to use EEG in clinical practice.

Primarily aimed at those who are in the earlier stages of using EEGs, this book offers a simpler overview that will offer a key resource to anyone using EEGs, no matter their level of experience.

T0133483

Making Sense of the EEG
From Basic Principles to Clinical Applications

Udaya Seneviratne

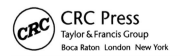

CRC Press
Taylor & Francis Group
Boca Raton London New York

CRC Press is an imprint of the
Taylor & Francis Group, an **informa** business

First edition published 2023
by CRC Press
6000 Broken Sound Parkway NW, Suite 300, Boca Raton, FL 33487-2742

and by CRC Press
4 Park Square, Milton Park, Abingdon, Oxon, OX14 4RN

CRC Press is an imprint of Taylor & Francis Group, LLC

ISBN: 9781032405537 (hbk)
ISBN: 9781032405407 (pbk)
ISBN: 9781003353713 (ebk)

DOI: 10.1201/9781003353713

Typeset in Minion Pro
by KnowledgeWorks Global Ltd.

Contents

Foreword

Interpretation of EEGs can be quite a challenge for neurology trainees – and indeed for many neurologists. Unlike electrocardiograms (ECGs), where even medical students achieve a basic level of competence, the collection, analysis, and interpretation of EEGs is foreign territory for most doctors. Further complicating this is the very wide range of normal variants and many "gray zones" between normal and abnormal patterns. The misinterpretation of normal patterns is a very significant problem in EEG reporting, often with significant impacts on patient management.

There are no contemporary Australian introductory texts on EEG – those available are generally directed to an audience that already has some basic understanding of the data while being comprehensive often overwhelming for the student. Professor Seneviratne has achieved with this work an excellent balance of practical information covering the basics of EEG acquisition through to the application of EEG in special settings such as ICU. Not intended as a comprehensive atlas, the work instead focuses on equipping the student with the essentials, moving on to the interpretation of normal patterns, and later various pathological states. Throughout, he provides excellent illustrations of the relevant waveforms.

As with his many publications in the field, the language is clear and precise, and the material is laid out in a logical and easy-to-follow manner. This work provides an excellent introduction to EEG, with all its complexities, in a readable and engaging form. I can highly recommend it to all students, and it should have a place on every aspiring neurologist's bookshelf!

Professor Mark Cook
MBBS, FRACP, MD, FRCP, FAAHMS

The Sir John Eccles Chair of Medicine, The University of Melbourne
Consultant Neurologist/Epileptologist & Director of Neurology
St. Vincent's Hospital Melbourne
Melbourne, Australia

Preface

The electroencephalogram (EEG) has become an indispensable tool in the investigation of epilepsies and several other neurological disorders. Therefore, EEG is an integral component of neurology training across the world. Though filled with intellectual excitement, reading EEGs can be a daunting task for a beginner. This book was inspired by my interactions with neurology advanced trainees in Australia during my supervision of EEG reading. Teaching them has provided me with a golden opportunity and privilege to understand their needs in learning EEGs efficiently, which formed the foundation of this book.

This publication is not meant to be a comprehensive textbook of EEG. My intention was to write a book that is easy to understand while providing a solid neurophysiological foundation to those who are in the early stages of their careers, including trainee neurologists, electroencephalographers, and EEG technologists. Hence, some neurophysiological concepts are presented in an oversimplified format for easy understanding by beginners.

This book starts with basic principles to educate the reader on the cellular and neurophysiological aspects as well as technical and engineering principles of EEG. It is followed by a section on normal EEG, and the next section covers the clinical applications of EEG in epilepsies and other brain disorders in detail. The final section is dedicated to critical care EEG, dealing with the most complex forms of EEG in clinical practice. Essentially, this book takes the reader on a journey, starting with basic principles followed by routine clinical applications and ending with the most difficult EEGs. Each chapter contains numerous figures of exemplar EEGs to help the reader understand the content easily. This book is designed to provide the reader with the necessary knowledge to use EEG in clinical practice and a good background knowledge of underpinning neurophysiologic principles. After reading this book, a beginner should feel confident to embark on their journey of interpreting EEGs.

I gratefully acknowledge my teachers, both direct and indirect in the form of published resources, for the knowledge I have acquired. I am indebted to EEG technologists who recorded the EEGs used as examples in the book. Lastly, I would like to thank my wife Rukmi and daughters Sinali and Tarini for their love and unwavering support in my academic endeavors.

Udaya Seneviratne
MBBS, MRCP (UK), FRACP, Ph.D.

Udaya Seneviratne, MBBS, MRCP (UK), FRACP, Ph.D., is an Associate Professor in Neurology and Epilepsy at The University of Melbourne. He is an Adjunct Clinical Associate Professor in Medicine at the School of Clinical Sciences at Monash Health, Monash University. In addition, Dr. Seneviratne is a consultant neurologist and epileptologist at Monash Medical Centre and St. Vincent's Hospital in Melbourne, Australia.

Section I

Basic principles

CHAPTER 1

The cellular and neurophysiological basis of EEG

Electroencephalograms (EEGs) are most often recorded noninvasively from the scalp. Semi-invasive EEG recordings involve nasopharyngeal and sphenoidal electrodes. Foramen ovale electrodes record from the extradural space close to the mesial temporal cortex. More invasive intracranial approaches include epidural, subdural, cortical, and intracerebral depth electrodes.

Electrocorticography involves the intraoperative recording of the EEG directly from the cortical surface. Stereoelectroencephalography (SEEG) as a method of depth recording is gaining more popularity due to its lower rate of complications and higher yield compared with subdural EEG recordings. This book will primarily focus on the scalp (surface) EEG.

In simple terms, EEG is a two-dimensional display of the activity occurring in the three-dimensional space of the brain. Two electrodes placed over the scalp measure the voltage difference between the two points. The voltage fluctuation is a dynamic process. When this voltage difference (y-axis) is plotted against time (x-axis), an EEG waveform is generated. Hence, the EEG provides the spatial resolution (based on the electrode distribution) as well as the temporal resolution. The challenge for the electroencephalographer is to solve the *inverse problem* of characterizing the intracerebral source based on the topography of the externally recorded EEG.

CELLULAR SOURCES OF EEG

The current understanding is that synaptic activity is the most significant contributor to the recorded EEG potentials. Neurons communicate with each other via synapses. When an action potential traveling through the axon reaches the presynaptic membrane, neurotransmitters are released from synaptic vesicles into the synaptic cleft. The response of the postsynaptic membrane depends on the neurotransmitter through its action on ion channels. When an excitatory neurotransmitter such as glutamate reaches the postsynaptic membrane, an influx of positively charged ions (usually Na^+) into the postsynaptic cell is triggered by a depolarization shift generating an excitatory postsynaptic potential (EPSP). On the contrary, inhibitory neurotransmitters (e.g., GABA) lead to efflux of positive ions (K^+) and/or influx of negative ions (Cl^-) across the postsynaptic membrane inducing hyperpolarization of the membrane and inhibitory postsynaptic potentials (IPSP). The summation of synchronous EPSP and IPSP generates cortical EEG waveforms.[1]

CORTICAL GENERATORS OF EEG

The cerebral cortex consists of six layers with the molecular layer I being the most superficial. The main generators of surface EEG are radially oriented cortical pyramidal neurons with cell bodies (soma) located in layer V and its vicinity.[2] As shown in Figure 1.1, there are four possible

DOI: 10.1201/9781003353713-2

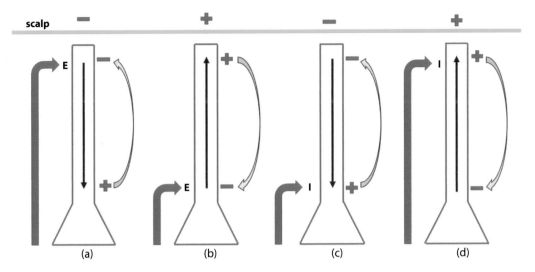

Figure 1.1 A schematic diagram to show the generation of EEG signals by cortical pyramidal neurons. The yellow arrow indicates the direction of the extracellular current while the red arrow represents the intracellular current flow. (a) An excitatory synapse (E) at the apical dendrite of the pyramidal cell results in an extracellular negative sink with a deeper positive source close to the soma. This activity generates a surface-negative wave on the scalp. (b) An excitatory synapse in a deep layer of the cortex creating a sink close to the soma and a dipole with surface positivity. (c) An inhibitory synapse (I) in a deep layer of the cortex creating a source close to the soma and a dipole with surface negativity. (d) An inhibitory synapse in a superficial layer of the cortex creating a source close to the surface and a dipole with surface positivity.

ways of generating surface-negative and surface-positive EEG waveforms, depending on the type of postsynaptic potential (EPSP versus IPSP) and the location of the synapse. When an EPSP is generated between an axonal terminal and an apical dendrite of the pyramidal neuron, that segment becomes electronegative extracellularly ("current sink") due to membrane depolarization. With that, the basal segment of the dendrite and the soma become electropositive ("current source") leading to current flow through the extracellular medium from the source to the sink. The result is a current dipole generating a surface-negative EEG waveform (Figure 1.1a). On the contrary, when the synapse and the resultant EPSP are located deeper, close to the soma, the polarity of the dipole is reversed, with the positive end facing the cortex, generating a surface-positive EEG waveform (Figure 1.1b). With IPSP, the exact opposite of this process is observed (Figure 1.1c & d).[3]

VOLUME CONDUCTION VERSUS PROPAGATION

The activity recorded from the scalp is the summation of two processes: volume conduction and propagation. Volume conduction is not energy-dependent whereas propagation is an energy-dependent active mechanism.[4,5] According to the volume conduction theory, the head is a three-dimensional volume conductor through which the electrical activity spreads from the generator instantaneously. The volume conduction is very fast, and an electrode located at a distant location will record the activity synchronous with the generator. While maintaining the original polarity and morphology, the waveform progressively attenuates in amplitude by a factor directly proportionate to the square of the distance from its generator.[6] On the contrary, with propagation, the waveform appears at a distant location after a time lag, but the polarity and the morphology may be distorted.[5] The time lag may not be obvious on cursory inspection, and the reader has to carefully study temporal relationships with an expanded timebase, special montages (reference-subtraction montage), or computer-aided analysis (Figure 1.2).[4] Propagation takes place through intracortical and subcortical neural pathways.

PRINCIPLES OF VOLUME CONDUCTION

The concept of the current dipole is the foundation of volume conduction theory. In the previous section on "Cortical Generators of EEG," we discussed the arrangement of cortical pyramidal neurons in the form of a current dipole with positive ("source") and negative ("sink") ends. In the most simplistic model, an epileptiform generator consists of thousands of pyramidal neurons lying parallel to each other, creating a composite dipole. The potential measured and recorded by a scalp electrode can be explained by the "solid angle" theory. The solid angle is an expression of the visible surface area of an object from a distant point. According to the solid angle theory, the potential recorded by the scalp electrode is directly proportional to the subtended solid angle at the electrode and the potential across the dipole layer.[7] For example, when we look at the moon from the earth, it appears very small as the subtended solid angle at the eye is small. However, an astronaut in a

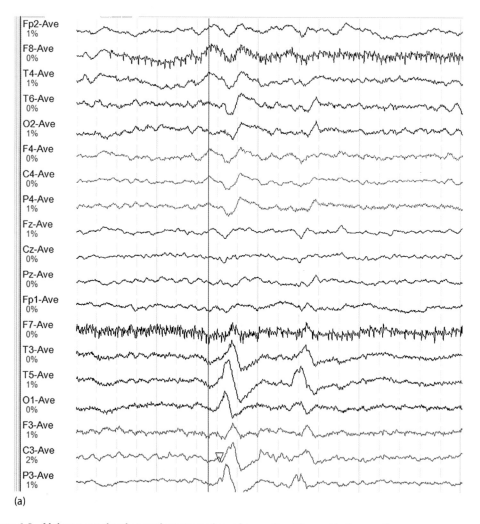

(a)

Figure 1.2   Volume conduction and propagation of an epileptiform discharge. Common average reference montage with (a) time base of 10 seconds per page, and (b) time base of 5 seconds per page. Note the voltage field created by volume conduction and propagation. The sharp wave with the highest amplitude is seen first on T5 indicating the "epicenter" of the field. Then, the field spreads to T3 O1, followed by P3 C3, and finally F3 electrodes. For each discharge, the time delay from the "epicenter" corresponds to propagation while amplitude reduction reflects volume conduction. *(Continued)*

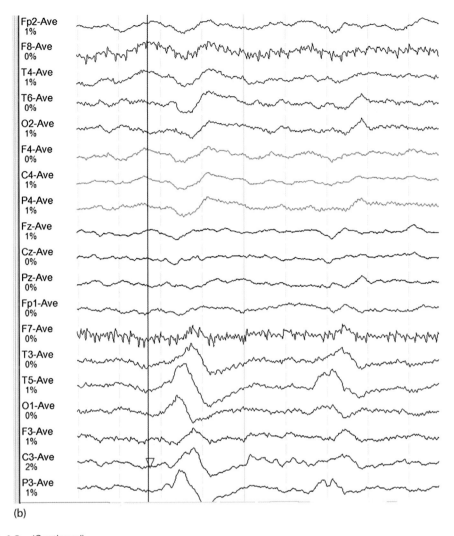

(b)

Figure 1.2 *(Continued)*

spacecraft approaching the moon will see it as a much larger object when the subtended solid angle increases. Based on the solid angle theory, it would be easy to resolve that an electrode that "sees" a larger area (with a larger solid angle) will record a higher potential. Similarly, an electrode "looking at" the negative end of the dipole will record a negative potential and vice versa. Therefore, we can deduce that the potential distribution (potential field) depends on the orientation of the dipole.[5,7]

Figure 1.3 shows a vertical (radial) dipole on the crown of a gyrus. The scalp electrode (e4) over the midpoint of the dipole enjoys the best "view" and has the widest solid angle, thus recording the highest potential. As the electrodes move away from the epicenter, the solid angle and the recorded potentials become smaller and smaller on either side (electrodes e3, e5). At points beyond e1 and e7, the solid angles and recorded potentials reach 0. The result is a voltage graph as shown in Figure 1.3. The figure shows how the gyrus and voltage graph appear on a coronal view, but it should be remembered that the dipole is in the three-dimensional space of the brain. Imagine you are looking at the head from above. In this bird's-eye view, you can connect points with the same potential and the outcome is an isopotential line. Multiple isopotential lines constitute a voltage field map as shown in the figure. Voltage fields are very useful to visualize where the maximum activity (epicenter) is and how it spreads. In a radial dipole of the human brain, we can visualize the voltage map for the negative pole only, as there are no electrodes placed on the positive pole.

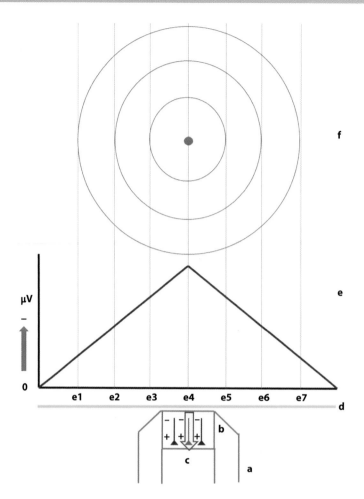

Figure 1.3 Schematic model of a radial dipole as well as the corresponding voltage graph and field map. (a) A cortical gyrus containing epileptogenic tissue (b) with numerous radially oriented pyramidal neurons and summation of activities generates a radially oriented equivalent current dipole (c). When electrodes (e1–e7) are placed on the scalp (d), the maximum potential is recorded by e4, which is directly above the dipole source subtending the highest solid angle. The voltage gradually declines on either side, as represented by the voltage graph (e). (f) The bird's-eye view of the voltage (isopotential) map generated by combining the points with the same potential (isopotential lines).

A horizontal dipole is likely to generate a different potential field. Such an orientation is possible when the source is on the wall of a sulcus (Figure 1.4). A horizontal dipole will generate both negative and positive fields on the scalp depending on the location of the electrode. The electrode (e4) overlying source "sees" both negative and positive ends of the dipole with equal solid angles neutralizing the potentials, and, as a result, recording 0. The electrodes e3 and e5 located away from the source have the best "views" of each end of the dipole, recording the maximum negative and positive potentials. The electrodes e1 and e7 at the extreme ends will also record much lower potentials. The outcome of the horizontal dipole is a symmetric sigmoid shape in the voltage graph. Looking from above, one can visualize the voltage field map by combining isopotential lines as explained under the radial dipole. In a horizontal dipole, it is possible to see both positive and negative voltage fields, as shown in Figure 1.4.

The third possible orientation is the oblique dipole (Figure 1.5). Such a generator will give rise to mostly negative potentials recorded from the surface accompanied by a small positive field, generating an asymmetric sigmoid shape in the voltage graph. The voltage field map will show a prominent negative field and a small positive field.

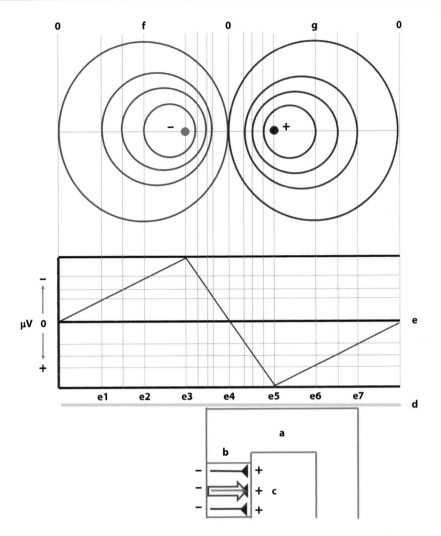

Figure 1.4 Schematic model of a horizontal dipole. A cortical gyrus is represented by (a) with an area of epileptogenic tissue (b) consisting of numerous pyramidal neurons aligned horizontal to the surface (d), generating negative and positive dipole layers. The summation of all individual dipoles is represented by (c). Seven electrodes (e1–e7) are placed on the scalp (d). E represents the voltage graph based on the potentials recorded at each electrode. The electrode e4 is at a right angle to the horizontal dipole and records 0 potential. The electrode e3 subtends the maximum solid angle "looking at" the negative end of the dipole, hence, recording the maximum negative activity. Similarly, e5 records the maximum positive activity. The orientation of the equivalent current dipole is depicted by the yellow arrow (c). (f and g) Bird's-eye views of the voltage field map seen on the surface that show the positive and negative ends of the dipole. The map is generated by combining spots with the same potential (isopotential lines). The zero isopotential line divides the positive and negative poles.

However, these theoretical concepts should be interpreted with caution due to many limitations. The dipole orientation may not be that straightforward, particularly in dysmorphic tissues.[5] Generators sometimes consist of multiple dipoles.[8] In the brain, volume conduction does not occur in a homogenous conductor. From the source to the scalp, different tissues have varying conductivities. As a result, the potentials recorded on the scalp become attenuated and fields may be distorted.[5]

It is an important practice tip to remember that the generator is not always underneath the electrode showing the maximum activity. It is the case in vertical dipoles, but with horizontal and oblique dipoles, the source is located away from the point recording the maximum activity on the scalp.

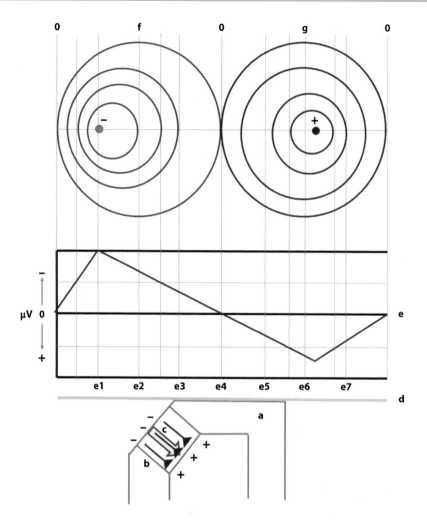

Figure 1.5 Schematic model of an oblique dipole. The bank of a cortical sulcus (a) has epileptogenic tissue (b) with obliquely oriented pyramidal neurons, generating an oblique dipole. In the voltage graph (e), the electrode e4 is at a right angle to the horizontal dipole and records 0 potential. The electrode e1 subtends the maximum solid angle "looking at" the negative end of the dipole, hence, recording the maximum negative activity. Similarly, e6 records the maximum positive activity (f and g). Bird's-eye views of the voltage field map seen on the surface that show the positive and the negative ends of the dipole.

FACTORS DETERMINING THE SCALP-RECORDED EEG ACTIVITY

With regard to the physical properties of the source, the location, area, orientation, and summation are the key factors influencing the EEG waveforms recorded from the scalp. To reach the surface electrode, the EEG activity must pass through several layers (inhomogeneous volume conductor). As a result, there is an attenuation of the activity based on the distance from the generator. To record from the scalp, the EEG activity has to be synchronized from a sufficient cortical area, which has been estimated to be a minimum of 6 cm².[1] However, subsequent research has revealed that a much larger area needs to be involved to capture interictal spikes and ictal rhythms.[9] As discussed in the previous section, the orientation of the dipole determines the type of potential field on the surface. When there are multiple adjacent cortical sources, the summated activity gives rise to the voltage field on the scalp. When multiple sources have the same orientation, the resultant voltage field is higher due to summation. On the contrary, when sources have different orientations, phase cancellation occurs and the final voltage field will reflect the sum of positive and negative vectors.

DIPOLE SOURCE MODELING

With the application of the principles of volume conduction, dipole source modeling is employed to solve the inverse problem, i.e., localizing the source based on the surface voltage field. To apply the principles of source modeling, one must define the appropriate source (point source versus distributed source), select a head model, and apply corrections for variable conductivities of the skull and the scalp. This section is not intended to be a detailed account of source modeling and analysis.

References

1. Cooper, R, Winter, AL, Crow, HJ, Walter, WG. Comparison of subcortical, cortical and scalp activity using chronically indwelling electrodes in man. Electroencephalogr Clin Neurophysiol 1965;18:217–228.

2. Ball, GJ, Gloor, P, Schaul, N. The cortical electromicrophysiology of pathological delta waves in the electroencephalogram of cats. Electroencephalogr Clin Neurophysiol 1977;43:346–361.

3. Mitzdorf, U. Current source-density method and application in cat cerebral cortex: Investigation of evoked potentials and EEG phenomena. Physiol Rev 1985;65:37–100.

4. Jayakar, P, Duchowny, MS, Resnick, TJ, Alvarez, LA. Localization of epileptogenic foci using a simple reference-subtraction montage to document small interchannel time differences. J Clin Neurophysiol 1991;8:212–215.

5. Jayakar, P, Duchowny, M, Resnick, TJ, Alvarez, LA. Localization of seizure foci: Pitfalls and caveats. J Clin Neurophysiol 1991;8:414–431.

6. Nunez, PL, Pilgreen, KL. The spline-Laplacian in clinical neurophysiology: A method to improve EEG spatial resolution. J Clin Neurophysiol 1991;8:397–413.

7. Gloor, P. Neuronal generators and the problem of localization in electroencephalography: Application of volume conductor theory to electroencephalography. J Clin Neurophysiol 1985;2:327–354.

8. Nunez, PL. The brain's magnetic field: Some effects of multiple sources on localization methods. Electroencephalogr Clin Neurophysiol 1986;63:75–82.

9. Ebersole, JS, Hawes-Ebersole, S. Clinical application of dipole models in the localization of epileptiform activity. J Clin Neurophysiol 2007;24:120–129.

CHAPTER 2

Principles of digital EEG recording and display

Digital electroencephalogram (EEG) recording consists of several steps involving a series of hardware and software. At least a basic understanding of this process is a must for all EEG readers to ensure optimal use of the available features and accurate interpretations. This chapter discusses the basic principles of digital EEG.

In brief, the voltage difference between two electrodes is amplified, filtered, digitized, and sent to a computer where EEG waveforms can be further manipulated with software and finally displayed. Figure 2.1 highlights those steps of a digital EEG system.

ELECTRODES

As mentioned in the previous chapter, electrodes capture the voltage on the surface and the EEG activity represents the voltage difference between two points captured by two electrodes. A "channel" is created when two electrodes are combined. The first electrode is called "input 1" (or active input) and the second electrode is "input 2." The channel displays a voltage equal to input 1 – input 2 (Figure 2.2a & b).

For optimum capture of this activity, good contact between the electrode and the scalp must be ensured. The "friction" or "resistance" between the two surfaces is expressed as impedance. It is recommended that at each scalp electrode, the impedance should be less than 5 kΩ. Higher impedances will increase the "noise" and introduce artifacts. Lower impedances are achieved by good skin preparation and application of an electrode gel or paste to improve contact. It is also important to achieve similar impedances at both inputs. Unusually low impedances (<100 Ω) should alert the technologist to look for bridging or short circuits (e.g., two electrodes connected by a salt bridge). Each electrode pair is also connected to a common ground electrode to minimize the 60 Hz electrostatic artifact (Figure 2.2a). In routine EEG recordings, the ground electrode is usually placed in the mid-forehead area. The ground electrode should not be confused with the "earth ground" of the EEG machine, an essential component of electrical safety. Conventional electrodes are usually made of platinum, gold, or silver-silver chloride. When multiple electrodes are used, as usually happens in EEG recording, it must be ensured that all electrodes are made of the same metal because inherent properties such as electrode potentials and time constants vary among different metals.

It is standard practice to place electrodes according to the "10–20 international system of electrode placement" to ensure consistency between different centers and serial recordings (Figure 2.3).[1] By convention, electrodes labeled with even numbers are placed on the right side and odd numbers on the left. The letters represent the anatomical location; F = frontal, Fp = frontopolar, T = temporal, P = parietal, O = occipital, and C = central. There are three electrodes on the sagittal midline from anterior to posterior (Fz, Cz, Pz). Figure 2.4 shows how these electrodes approximately correspond to different brain regions.

    DOI: 10.1201/9781003353713-3

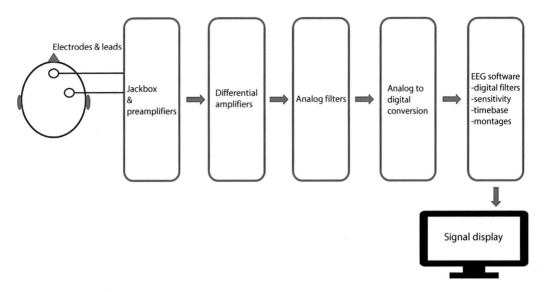

Figure 2.1   Schematic diagram showing the key steps in digital EEG recording and display.

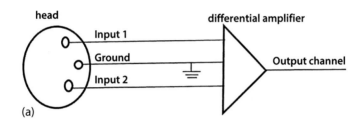

Input 1		Input 2		Output (input1 – input2)	
−10		−10		0	
−10		+10		−20	
−20		−10		−10	
+10		−10		+20	

(b)

Figure 2.2   How electrodes are combined for EEG recording. (a) Two electrode inputs connected via an amplifier give rise to an output channel. The ground connection is common to all electrode derivations. (b) Schematic diagram showing the relationship between the two inputs and the output. Please note the output is shown without amplification for easy understanding (input 1 – input 2 = output). In reality, after going through the amplifier, the output voltage is equal to (input 1 – input 2) × amplification factor.

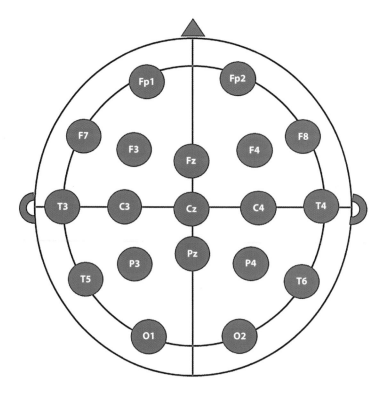

Figure 2.3   The 10–20 international system of electrode placement.

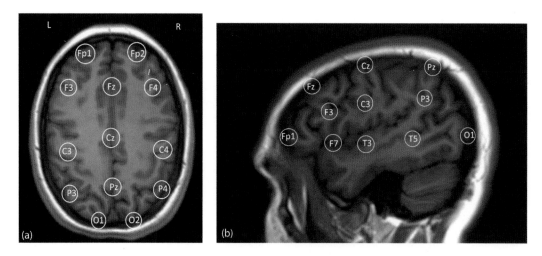

Figure 2.4   Approximate electrode positions in relation to brain regions. (a) axial view; (b) left lateral view.

As mentioned, two inputs are needed to acquire EEG signals. In digital EEG, all signal acquisitions occur using a common "machine reference electrode (recording reference)" as the input 2. The machine (recording) reference should not be mistaken for the ground reference electrode described at the beginning of this section. The machine reference is placed in an area least susceptible to artifacts, usually on the central midline. In the montage for signal acquisition, each channel consists of an active input (input 1) and a common input (input 2, machine reference electrode). For each channel, each individual electrode of 10–20 placement becomes input 1. This montage ensures signal acquisition from all the electrodes. After digitization, this data can be easily reformatted by the EEG software into multiple different montages at the time of EEG reading.

JACKBOX

The jackbox is essentially a board with sockets providing space to plug in the electrode pins. It is usually labeled in keeping with the international 10–20 system, and the terminal end of the electrode extension wire can be plugged into the appropriate slot. The standard EEG usually has 32 electrode inputs, but jackboxes of modern EEG machines can accommodate a higher number of inputs (such as 256) to facilitate multi-channel and high-density EEG recordings. Additionally, multiple polygraphic channels such as EMG, ECG, and oximetry can also be connected to the jackbox. Usually, they are connected to a meter to measure the impedance without unplugging the electrode.

AMPLIFIERS

There are two major challenges to overcome in recording EEG signals. The potentials captured at the scalp level are very small (in microvolts) and to render them "visible," the signals have to be "enlarged." The second challenge is the background noise. The EEG recordings take place in an environment full of electrical "noise" due to electrical wiring and mains-operated equipment generating electrostatic and electromagnetic fields that cause interference. These two challenges are overcome using amplifiers.

The key functions of amplifiers are amplification and common-mode rejection. Differential amplifiers can achieve those objectives. As shown in Figure 2.2, the amplifier receives two inputs. The voltage difference between the two inputs (input 1 – input 2) is amplified. The amplified output is equal to the voltage difference between the two inputs multiplied by a constant known as *Gain*. Gain is usually expressed in decibels as a logarithmic ratio of output voltage divided by the input voltage (gain = $20 \times \log$ [output voltage/input voltage]). The degree of amplification achieved by a single amplifier is usually not sufficient. Hence, to increase the total gain, a series of amplifiers linked together is used in EEG machines.

The second important function is common-mode rejection. Similar potentials going through both inputs are called common-mode signals whereas different potentials are termed differential-mode signals. Common modes are removed from the output due to subtraction and this phenomenon is known as "common-mode rejection." As a result, amplifiers can eliminate unwanted noise such as the 50 Hz artifact. The common-mode rejection ratio (CMMR) is an expression of the amplifier's ability to display differential-mode signals while attenuating common-mode signals. CMMR is equal to the gain of the differential-mode signal divided by the gain of the common-mode signal and usually expressed in decibels after logarithmic transformation: CMMR = $20 \times \log_{10}$ (differential-mode gain/common-mode gain). The American Clinical Neurophysiology Society (ACNS) recommends CMMR of ≥ 90 dB.[2] It should be noted that even in-phase biological signals are also eliminated by common-mode rejection due to phase cancellation (Chapter 3, Figure 3.1c).

Electromagnetic fields in the environment can induce currents in the loop involving the patient, electrodes, leads, and the amplifier generating voltage differences between the electrodes. To minimize this interference, EEG amplifiers are designed with high input impedances. The amplifier input impedance should not be mistaken for electrode impedance, which should be kept low to reduce noise. Maintaining equal impedances across electrodes, and keeping the electrode leads short and bundled together are other ways to minimize interference. The first amplifier (preamplifier) in the system is usually located in the jackbox. Each electrode input has its own preamplifier. Preamplifiers capture the source signal while minimizing the interference significantly, so that subsequent differential amplifiers can boost the signal adequately and efficiently.

FILTERS

The signals captured by the electrodes are a mixture of EEG frequencies we are interested in as well as unwanted "noise." Filters are used to attenuate the noise and separate EEG signals based on their frequencies so that we can focus on the EEG activity. In digital EEG machines, filtering occurs at two stages—before digitization and after digitization. Analog filters used during pre-digitization are hardwired into the machine, whereas digital filters are part of the computer software that facilitates reformatting and reprocessing of the data after the signal acquisition and digitization.

According to the frequency bands allowed through, filters can be categorized into four groups.

1. *Low-frequency filter (LFF):* This is also called the high-pass filter. This filter allows frequencies above the cutoff frequency to pass through while attenuating slower frequencies below the cutoff. The main function of LFF is to remove slow direct current (DC) potentials and artifacts.

2. *High-frequency filter (HFF):* This type is also known as the low-pass filter and has the opposite action of LFF. HFF allows all frequencies below the cutoff limit to pass through while attenuating frequencies above the cutoff.

3. *Band-pass filter:* This filter allows frequencies between upper and lower cutoff values to pass through while attenuating all other frequencies.

4. *Band-stop or notch filter:* This filter attenuates frequencies within a narrow range while allowing frequencies above and below the range to pass through. The main function of the notch filter in the EEG machine is to remove 50 or 60 Hz interference from the power supply. However, the appearance of the 50 Hz artifact during the EEG recording alerts the technologists regarding faults. If the 50 Hz artifact appears in a channel during the recording, it indicates a high impedance of the particular electrode, which needs to be corrected. The appearance of the 50 Hz artifact in all channels during the recording usually suggests high impedances of the ground or reference electrodes or faulty grounding of the EEG machine, which requires urgent attention. For this reason, the notch filter should be open (or turned off) during data acquisition.[3] It is good practice to review the EEG at the beginning of the recording, with the machine reference montage to detect high impedances of electrodes, and, particularly, the machine reference electrode so that it can be rectified early. If any 50 Hz activity is captured, it can be eliminated post-digitization using the notch filter of the software. However, signal loss due to faulty electrodes cannot be rectified after data acquisition.

We probably visualize an abrupt cutoff at the set frequency limit when filters are applied. On the contrary, filters demonstrate a gradual transition with attenuation of output amplitude on either side of the cutoff frequency.

Conventional EEG recording involves LFF of 0.1 Hz and HFF of 100 Hz at the time of signal acquisition. This bandwidth generally captures EEG frequencies we analyze in routine practice. However, it excludes infraslow activity and fast high-frequency oscillations that may provide additional valuable information, particularly concerning epileptiform activity. The value of "full-band" or "wideband" EEG to capture these very slow and very fast frequencies has been discussed by researchers.[4] It is important to remember that only acquired signals can be reprocessed with digital filters after analog-to-digital conversion. If an electroencephalographer wants to study high-frequency oscillations, those signals should be captured during the stage of data acquisition by applying the appropriate filter settings.

A special and important type of HFF applied before digitization is the antialiasing filter. This filter attenuates higher frequencies to reduce the possibility of signal aliasing. The concept of aliasing will be discussed in detail in the next section.

ANALOG-TO-DIGITAL CONVERSION

The analog to digital conversion of signals through a digitizing circuit is a crucial step. Analog signals appear as a continuous line with continuously changing values across the time scale. To digitize, the analog signal must be sampled multiple times in two independent axes (time and amplitude) and processed.

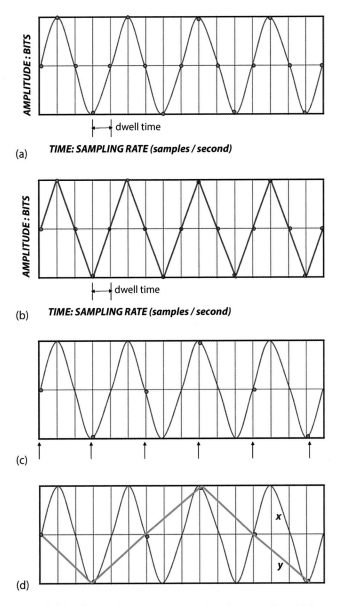

Figure 2.5 Principles of digitization and consequences of undersampling. (a) An analog signal of a sine wave (4 Hz frequency) spread over 1 second and ready for digitization. (b) The digitized signal of the sine wave at a sampling rate of 16/second. Note the outcome is a wave with similar morphology and an identical frequency of 4 Hz. (c) The same analog sine wave ready for digitization at a lower sampling rate (5.3/second). (d) The outcome (y) has little resemblance to the original analog signal (x) with a much lower frequency. This phenomenon is called aliasing.

Let's first look at the sampling along the time axis. Figure 2.5a shows an analog signal of a sine wave recurring at 4 Hz. We take measurements at regular intervals. Each measurement is called a sample. The sampling interval (also called dwell time) is the time gap between two successive samples. The number of samples per second, measured in hertz, is called the sampling rate (sampling rate = 1 / sampling interval). Figure 2.5b shows the digital signal generated at the current sampling rate of 16 Hz. This waveform has a reasonable similarity to the original analog signal with the same frequency. When the sampling rate is increased, the digital signal gains more resemblance to the original analog waveform. Let's see what happens when the sampling rate is reduced to 5.3 Hz (Figure 2.5c) and the result is a distorted signal with poor or no resemblance to the original waveform (Figure 2.5d).

This phenomenon is called "aliasing," which is a considerable problem caused by undersampling during digitization resulting in spurious digital signals. It is clear that higher sampling rates will generate better resolution, but will require more storage space with larger files. Hence comes the question "what is the optimal sampling rate?" The Nyquist theorem posits that the sampling rate must be at least twice the frequency to be digitized. This minimum sampling rate is called the Nyquist rate and the corresponding frequency of the signal being digitized is known as Nyquist frequency.[5] For example, if the EEG recording system has a sampling rate of 200 (Nyquist rate), the highest frequency that can be digitized by the system is 100 Hz (Nyquist frequency). The ACNS recommends a sampling rate of more than three times the HFF setting and higher rates are preferred for better resolution and automated spike detection.[2] Most EEG systems offer sampling rates of 256 Hz or more. Aliasing occurs when the sampling rate is less than the Nyquist rate.[5] Aliasing should be prevented at the time of EEG signal acquisition by selecting an appropriate sampling rate and the use of an antialiasing filter. The antialiasing filter should be selected in keeping with the sampling rate to attenuate frequencies above the Nyquist frequency. Aliasing is not correctable later with data reprocessing.

The other part of digitization occurs along the amplitude (vertical) axis. The amplitude is divided into several levels and expressed in terms of bits. Each bit is a power of two and the higher the bit number the better the amplitude resolution. For example, 3 bits are equal to eight levels or divisions (2^3). Figure 2.6 illustrates this concept. Imagine a sine wave with an amplitude of 800 µV. With 3 bit resolution, this 800 µV is spread over eight levels (divisions), indicating each level is 100 µV. When the signal is digitized, values within each level (0–99) will not show any variation. However, when it reaches the next level, a stepwise change occurs. Therefore, large amplitude changes within a level can be undetected while small changes between levels are overrepresented. This can be overcome by increasing the bit resolution. When the bit resolution is increased to 4, an 800 µV wave is spread across 16 levels, providing a much better resolution of 50 µV per level.

The ACNS recommends a resolution of 16 bits or more.[2] If the depth is 16 bits, the signal is vertically spread across 65,536 levels (2^{16}). If we record a wave with an amplitude of 800 µV, the amplitude resolution will be 0.0122 µV (800/65,536).

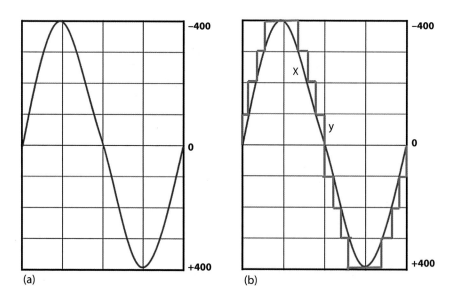

Figure 2.6 A schematic diagram of digitization along the vertical axis. (a) This analog signal of a sine wave with an amplitude of 800 µV is ready for digitization across eight divisions along the amplitude axis. (b) The outcome with digitization (y) in comparison to the analog signal (x). Note stepwise change in amplitude as explained in the text.

REFORMATTING OF EEG SIGNALS WITH COMPUTER SOFTWARE

The option of reformatting data after the acquisition is a major advantage of the digital EEG over analog recordings. In analog EEG, once the technologist has completed the record, the reader can only study the data as presented. On the other hand, digital EEG provides the opportunity for the electroencephalographer to reformat the data in many ways for better display and interpretation of the results. However, in this process, the electroencephalographer should be careful to avoid potential pitfalls inherently associated with digital reformatting. This reformatting is possible in several domains such as filters, sensitivity, montages, and time scale. Digital EEG also provides opportunities for automated analysis (artifact identification, spike, and seizure detection), topographic mapping, source modeling, and quantitative EEG. We will be primarily focusing on digital reformatting in this chapter.

Filters

Digital filters are designed to attenuate unwanted "noise" while retaining the "signals" we are interested in studying. This process invariably causes signal distortion and filter artifacts. Hence, one must give careful consideration before applying filters and the outcomes must be interpreted with caution. Despite those limitations, digital filtering is an important step in EEG reading and rational application of filtering enhances EEG interpretation. Systematic inspection of both the unfiltered and filtered signals is recommended to identify signal distortions and recognize signal elements removed by the filtering process.[6]

Finite impulse response (FIR) and infinite impulse response (IIR) filters are commonly used in digital EEG systems.[7] IIR filters are fast, requiring less computing power, but are relatively unstable and more susceptible to signal distortions. FIR filters require more computational power but are more stable with fewer distortions.

When reading the EEG, the electroencephalographer has the option to change the settings of HFF and LFF. Additionally, if the 50 Hz artifact is visible, the notch filter can be applied. All these options are incorporated into the EEG reading software. The electroencephalographer should change the filter settings rationally to optimize EEG interpretation while avoiding potential pitfalls.

Lowering the HFF may be useful to unmask underlying EEG rhythms when there is too much noise created by high-frequency muscle artifacts. However, the reader must be mindful of pitfalls due to data loss. Fast frequencies of cerebral origin, including epileptiform discharges, may be filtered off and disappear from the screen. Furthermore, not all muscle activity is filtered off and the remaining artifact may resemble beta rhythm, which can be misinterpreted by a novice EEG reader (also read Chapter 7).

When the EEG is contaminated with low-frequency artifacts such as movement and sweat artifacts, elevating the LFF may eliminate those unwanted slow waves (Figure 2.7a & b). However, the downside is the loss of slow frequencies of cerebral origin such as slow-wave of the spike and wave complex.

Sensitivity

The amplitude of the waveform we visualize depends on the sensitivity, which is equal to the ratio between the input voltage and output deflection. Often, in routine EEG readings, the sensitivity is set to 7–10 μV/mm. The sensitivity of 10 μV/mm means 1 mm deflection on the screen represents an input of 10 μV. Higher numerical values of sensitivity indicate lower amplification of the waveform. The reader is at liberty to change the sensitivity to study the EEG waveforms better. For example, waveforms of high amplitude at 7 μV/mm may overlap, making it harder to study morphology. Changing the sensitivity to a higher numerical value of 30 μV/mm (or lowering amplification) will reduce the display amplitude (Figure 2.8a & b). Conversely, if the amplitude is too low, increasing the magnification by setting the sensitivity at a lower value can be helpful.

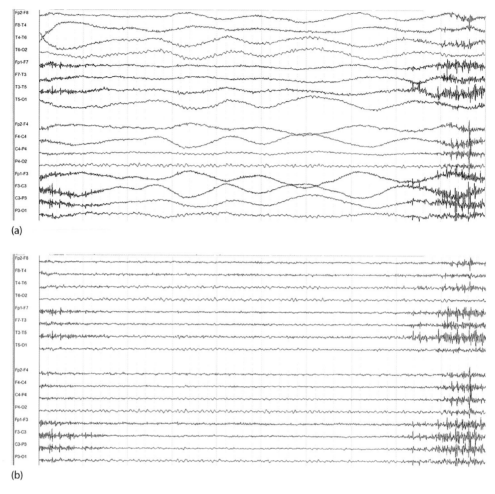

(a)

(b)

Figure 2.7   Removal of low-frequency artifacts by changing the low-frequency filter. (a) A low-frequency artifact due to sweat making it difficult to appreciate the background (high-frequency filter = 70 Hz, low-frequency filter = 0.5 Hz) (b) Same EEG epoch with the low-frequency filter set to 3 Hz to remove the artifact.

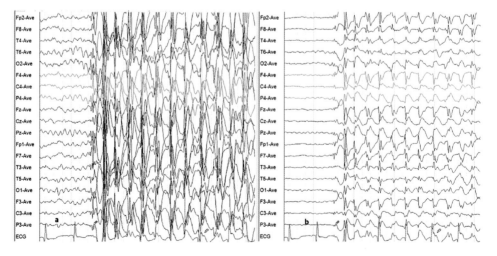

Figure 2.8   Changing the display sensitivity to study waveform frequency and morphology. (a) An absence seizure displayed at 10 μV/mm. Due to the high amplitude of overlapping waveforms, it is difficult to appreciate the frequency and morphology of the activity. (b) The same EEG epoch with the sensitivity set to 40 μV/mm. With lowered amplitude, it is easier to study the waveforms in detail.

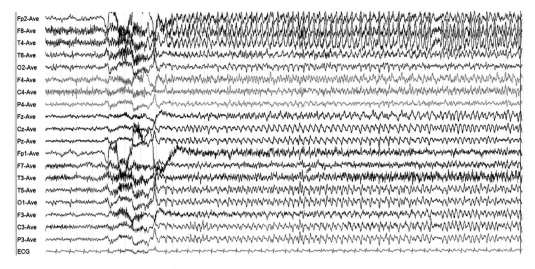

Figure 2.9 Evolving ictal rhythm of a right temporal seizure in a patient with right hippocampal sclerosis displayed with the timebase compressed to 30 sec/page.

Timebase

In the analog EEG, the timebase is determined by the paper speed, which usually is 30 mm/second. However, with digital EEG, the reader can change the timebase and decide how many seconds of the EEG record are displayed as one "page" (or one epoch) on the computer screen. When you look at the EEG, the distance between two vertical lines represents 1 second. Most often, readers tend to choose 10 seconds per page (epoch).

Compressing the timebase (e.g., 30 seconds/page) is helpful to screen the EEG quickly. Additionally, periodic activity is better visualized with a compressed timebase. Another use is to elicit evolving ictal rhythms (Figure 2.9). However, waveform morphologies become less discernible when the timebase is compressed.

Expanding the timebase can help to demonstrate complex morphologies and spatial-temporal relationships (Chapter 1, Figure 1.2a & b). It can assist the reader to determine the electrode of likely ictal onset in an electrographic seizure. Fast EEG frequencies can be accurately counted by expanding the time base to 1 second/page.

Montages

As we have discussed, two electrodes join to make a channel and when multiple channels are joined in a logical order, a montage is created. Montages are used to make EEG reading easier, more effective, and more accurate. The main advantage of digital over analog EEG is the ability to re-montage, which is made possible by the way EEG signals are acquired. In digital EEG, the signal acquisition of all electrodes (input 1) is achieved in relation to a common reference electrode (input 2). As a result, any montage can be re-created after the recording is completed.

Based on how electrodes are connected, there are two main categories of montages: bipolar and referential. In a bipolar montage, electrode pairs are linked in the form of a chain whereby the second input of each channel becomes the first input of the next channel. Conversely, in a referential montage, all channels have a common (reference) input 2. There are several types of referential montages based on what constitutes input 2 (or the reference electrode). Rules of localization will be discussed in Chapter 3, but in brief, in a bipolar montage, localization depends on phase reversal whereas amplitude is the key feature assisting localization in a referential montage.

Bipolar montage

Electrode pairs are linked across transverse, longitudinal, or circumferential lines in a bipolar montage (Figure 2.10). The longitudinal bipolar montage is also popularly known as "double-banana montage" due to its shape. Each electrode chain can be arranged by hemisphere or alternating from side to side (Table 2.1).

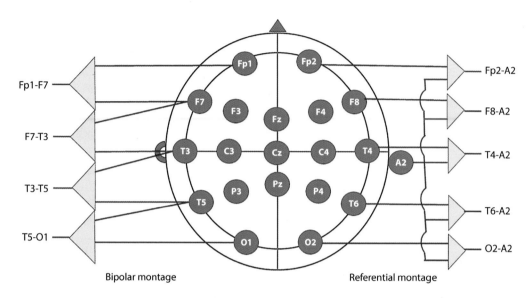

Figure 2.10   How electrodes are linked in longitudinal bipolar montage and ear reference montage. Only the most lateral electrode derivations are shown here for simplicity.

Table 2.1   Some examples of bipolar montages

Channel	Longitudinal bipolar: Right to left alternating	Longitudinal bipolar: Hemispheric	Transverse bipolar
1	Fp2–F4	Fp2–F8	F8–Fp2
2	F4–C4	F8–T4	Fp2–Fp1
3	C4–P4	T4–T6	Fp1–F7
4	P4–O2	T6–O2	F8–F4
5	Fp1–F3	Fp2–F4	F4–Fz
6	F3–C3	F4–C4	Fz–F3
7	C3–P3	C4–P4	F3–F7
8	P3–O1	P4–O2	A2–T4
9	Fz–Cz	Fz–Cz	T4–C4
10	Cz–Pz	Cz–Pz	C4–Cz
11	Fp2–F8	Fp1–F3	Cz–C3
12	F8–T4	F3–C3	C3–T3
13	T4–T6	C3–P3	T3–A1
14	T6–O2	P3–O1	T6–P4
15	Fp1–F7	Fp1–F7	P4–Pz
16	F7–T3	F7–T3	Pz–P3
17	T3–T5	T3–T5	P3–T5
18	T5–O1	T5–O1	T6–O2
19			O2–O1
20			O1–T5

The longitudinal bipolar montage is a good option for screening the EEG to study the background and spot abnormalities by way of phase reversal. Phase reversal occurs at the point of maximum voltage in any bipolar montage. Due to its unique electrode linking, bipolar montage is ideal to search for "needles in a haystack." A waveform of low amplitude with a narrow voltage field buried in a background of high-amplitude potentials is difficult to identify on a referential montage. When a bipolar montage is used, widely distributed high-amplitude waveforms are canceled out (in-phase cancellation, see Chapter 3, Figure 3.1c) and small potentials with a narrow field stand out for easy detection. The transverse bipolar montage is particularly useful to visualize sleep potentials and midline potentials.

However, bipolar montages are not without limitations. Widely distributed background potentials attenuate due to in-phase cancellation. For the same reason, an isopotential line ("flatline") does not mean the absence of EEG activity. It simply indicates that both inputs 1 and 2 of the channel have identical potentials. Remember, channel output = input 1 − input 2. In a wide field, the adjoining channels can be isopotential. This appearance can be misread by an inexperienced beginner. Another limitation is the "end of chain phenomenon" where no phase reversal occurs to help localization when the voltage maximum is at or beyond the first or last electrode of the chain (Chapter 3, Figure 3.7). Furthermore, bipolar montage is not suitable to study the amplitude, asymmetry, morphology, synchrony, or voltage fields of waveforms. Less commonly, "out-of-phase augmentation" may give rise to waveforms of spuriously high voltage when two electrodes with opposite polarities are combined to form a channel (Chapter 3, Figure 3.1f).[8]

Common reference montage

In this montage, each individual electrode (input 1) is combined with a common reference electrode (input 2). The options for reference electrodes include the ipsilateral ear (A1, A2) and Cz (Figure 2.10 and Table 2.2).[9] The main requirement for the reference electrode is to be "neutral" or "quiet." In other words, the reference electrode should be located outside the voltage field of interest

Table 2.2   Some examples of referential montages

Channel	Ear reference: Hemispheric	Cz reference: Right to left alternating	Cz reference: Hemispheric
1	F8–A2	F8–Cz	F8–Cz
2	T4–A2	F7–Cz	T4–Cz
3	T6–A2	T4–Cz	T6–Cz
4	Fp2–A2	T3–Cz	Fp2–Cz
5	F4–A2	T6–Cz	F4–Cz
6	C4–A2	T5–Cz	C4–Cz
7	P4–A2	Fp2–Cz	P4–Cz
8	O2–A2	Fp1–Cz	O2–Cz
9	Fz–A2	F4–Cz	Fz–Cz
10	Cz–A2	F3–Pz	Pz–Cz
11	Pz–A2	C4–Cz	Fp1–Cz
12	Fp1–A1	C3–Cz	F3–Cz
13	F3–A1	P4–Cz	C3–Cz
14	C3–A1	P3–Cz	P3–Cz
15	P3–A1	O2–Cz	O1–Cz
16	O1–A1	O1–Cz	F7–Cz
17	F7–A1	Fz–Cz	T3–Cz
18	T3–A1	Pz–Cz	T5–Cz
19	T5–A1		

to avoid "reference contamination." The second rule is to choose an electrode with minimal or no artifacts and prominent physiological graphoelements, such as sleep activity.

The localization in the common reference montage is based on the amplitude. Contrary to the bipolar montage, the reference montage is very useful to study amplitude, asymmetry, morphology, and voltage fields. It is a better option than the bipolar montage to display phase relationships and widespread activities. Propagating activity is best displayed on this montage provided a suitable "neutral" reference electrode is chosen away from the field.

To display generalized EEG activities with widespread fields, such as generalized spike-wave discharges, generalized rhythmic delta activity, and generalized triphasic waves, ipsilateral ear reference is a good option. However, an inherent drawback of ear reference is contamination with the temporalis muscle and ECG artifacts. Ipsilateral ear reference should not be used to study fields involving the temporal lobe (e.g., temporal sharp waves) as the reference electrodes are in the field of interest. Due to in-phase cancellation, spurious phase reversals and fields may be generated, which can be misleading. Ear reference is suitable to study an anterior frontal focus as the field is remote from the reference electrode.

Cz reference is a reasonable alternative to studying narrow temporal fields. The main drawback is contamination with sleep activity (e.g., vertex waves) as the state changes.

Common average reference montage

The common average reference montage is created by devising a reference electrode to display EEG activity uniformly in a predictable and easily interpretable format. This is achieved by obtaining the average voltage of all electrodes in any given instance to serve as input 2. If the montage is reliable, at any given time point, the sum of deflections (positive and negative) from all channels should be zero. A major drawback of this montage is that localized high-amplitude activity, either cerebral or artifactual, will "bias" reference in that direction, generating spurious waveforms of opposite polarity in other channels. One good example is the impact of eye blinks (Figure 2.11). To minimize the impact of eye blinks and eye movements, frontopolar, and anterior temporal electrodes (Fp1, Fp2, F7, F8) can be excluded when creating the average reference.[9]

The common average reference is a great option to detect discrete foci with narrow fields, but it can also display diffuse activity reasonably well. Studying polarity, asymmetry, amplitude, voltage field, and phase relations between electrodes are other applications of this montage.

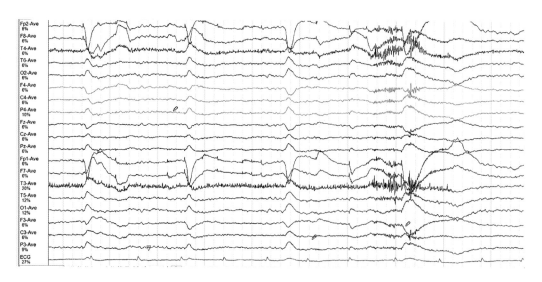

Figure 2.11   Effect of eye blinks on common average reference montage.

Source derivation (Laplacian) montage

This is a unique montage in creating a reference for each electrode (input 1) by using the weighted average of surrounding electrodes. As opposed to the common average reference that uses the average of all electrodes as the reference, Laplacian montage creates multiple "local (weighted) averages" for each input 1 to enhance the spatial resolution. It works best with high-density EEG with more electrodes. The source localization is based on the amplitude criteria, similar to referential montages.

Laplacian montage is an excellent option to display well-localized focal activity. However, when the field is large and diffuse, the peripheral activity is attenuated while displaying the voltage maxima prominently to create a false impression of a narrow field (Figure 2.12a & b).

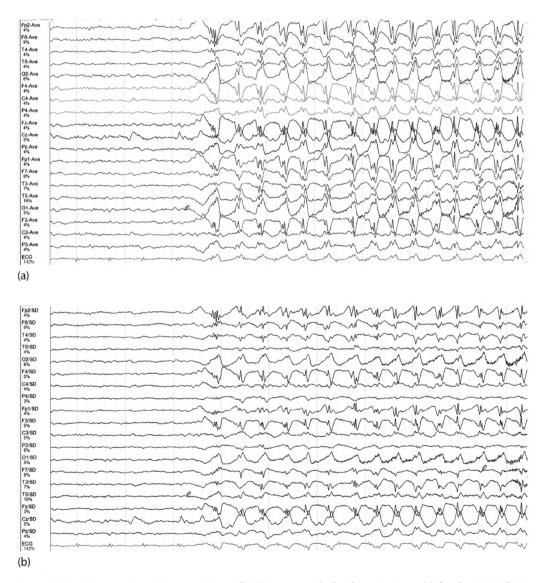

(a)

(b)

Figure 2.12   Attenuation of the peripheral field in source derivation montage. (a) An absence seizure displayed on the common average reference montage. Note the field maxima in fronto-central regions spreading to the periphery with a gradual lowering of amplitudes. (b) The same EEG epoch displayed on the source derivation montage. The fronto-central maxima are still clearly visible. However, there is considerable attenuation of the activity in the peripheral temporal and parietal regions giving the impression of a much smaller field compared with (a).

Table 2.3 summarizes a comparison of different practical applications among montages.

Table 2.3   Strengths and weaknesses of commonly used montages

	Bipolar	Common reference*	Common average reference	Source derivation
Localization is based on	Phase reversal	Amplitude	Amplitude	Amplitude
Display of background rhythm	Good	Good	Fair	Fair
Display of focal activity	Good	Good	Good Poor—if the background is high amplitude	Good
Display of generalized activity with a broad field	Poor	Good	Fair	Poor
Display of focal attenuation	Poor	Good	Fair	Poor
Display of propagating waves	Poor	Good	Fair	Fair
Display of asymmetry	Poor	Good	Good—focal asymmetry Poor—widespread asymmetry	Fair
Display of dipoles	Poor	Good	Fair	Fair
Display of amplitudes	Poor	Good	Good	Good
Display of morphology	Poor—generalized activity Fair—focal activity	Good	Good—focal Fair—generalized	Good—focal Fair—generalized
Display of topography/ voltage fields	Poor	Good	Good—focal Fair—generalized	Good—focal Poor—generalized
Localization of electrode and lead artifacts	Good	Good	Poor—high amplitude artifact Fair—others	Fair

Note:
* Assumption here is that a proper "neutral" reference is selected.

SIGNAL DISPLAY

The most versatile method is to display the digital signals on a computer screen. It is important to ensure the monitor has sufficient temporal and spatial resolution for an accurate signal display. The resolution is expressed in terms of pixels. As described below, aliasing can occur at the level of signal display, and digital antialiasing filters incorporated into the software are designed to minimize the impact.

Horizontal resolution

The temporal resolution is represented horizontally. The ACNS recommends a minimum horizontal screen resolution of 1,280 pixels for a 10-second page (128 pixels/second) whilst 1 second should correspond to 25–35 mm on the horizontal axis.[2] Therefore, how much data can be displayed on a screen depends on the number of pixels the screen embodies.

Analogous to the Nyquist theorem, the maximum frequency that can be reliably displayed on a screen is equal to 50% of the number of pixels per second on the horizontal axis.[10] This means a minimum of two pixels is required to display a waveform of 1 Hz frequency. Any waveform with a frequency of more than half the pixel resolution of the screen is susceptible to aliasing on display.[10] Let's consider a computer screen with 1,280 pixels on the horizontal axis. If 280 pixels are occupied by montage labels on the left side of the screen, only 1,000 pixels are available to display the EEG data. If you display an EEG epoch of 10 seconds on the screen, the resolution is 100 pixels/second and any waveform >50 Hz may not be displayed clearly. Higher frequencies may be spuriously displayed as slower frequencies and this error can be corrected by changing the display window to a higher pixel rate (e.g., 5 second epoch = 200 pixels/second) or switching to a monitor with a higher resolution.[10]

Vertical Resolution

Similar to horizontal resolution, the limiting factors are the pixel resolution and height of the screen. The vertical resolution of ≥4 pixels/mm and ≥10 mm per channel display is recommended.[2,3] Let's imagine an EEG displayed with 8 µV/mm sensitivity on a monitor with 4 pixels/mm screen resolution. This resolution means one pixel is equal to 0.25 mm of the screen height representing 2 µV of activity. If this EEG has a waveform with an amplitude of 1 µV, it will be displayed as a flat line rather than a waveform as it occupies less than one pixel vertically. If we change the display sensitivity to 2 µV/mm, the equation changes. Now, one pixel is equal to 0.25 mm of the screen height representing 0.5 µV of activity which means there are two pixels vertically representing 1 µV and the waveform becomes "visible" on display. This is the reason why we need to choose a monitor with adequate height and pixels for optimum signal display.

There are many exemplar EEGs throughout this book to help the reader understand the content and recognize patterns. These EEGs are usually displayed with LFF 0.5 Hz, HFF 70 Hz, sensitivity 10 µV/mm, and timebase 10 sec/page. Whenever there is deviation from the usual settings, it will be specified in the figure legend.

References

1. Jasper, HH. Report of the committee on methods of clinical examination in electroencephalography: 1957. Electroencephalogr Clin Neurophysiol 1958;10:370–375.

2. Halford, JJ, Sabau, D, Drislane, FW, Tsuchida, TN, Sinha, SR. American Clinical Neurophysiology Society guideline 4: Recording clinical EEG on digital media. J Clin Neurophysiol 2016;33:317–319.

3. Seneviratne, U. Rational manipulation of digital EEG: Pearls and pitfalls. J Clin Neurophysiol 2014;31:507–516.

4. Vanhatalo, S, Voipio, J, Kaila, K. Full-band EEG (FbEEG): An emerging standard in electroencephalography. Clin Neurophysiol 2005;116:1–8.

5. Nilsson, J, Panizza, M, Hallett, M. Principles of digital sampling of a physiologic signal. Electroencephalogr Clin Neurophysiol 1993;89:349–358.

6. Widmann, A, Schroger, E, Maess, B. Digital filter design for electrophysiological data–A practical approach. J Neurosci Methods 2015;250:34–46.

7. Cook, EW, Miller, GA. Digital filtering: Background and tutorial for psychophysiologists. Psychophysiology 1992;29:350–367.

8. Jayakar, P, Duchowny, M, Resnick, TJ, Alvarez, LA. Localization of seizure foci: Pitfalls and caveats. J Clin Neurophysiol 1991;8:414–431.

9. Acharya, JN, Hani, AJ, Thirumala, PD, Tsuchida, TN. American Clinical Neurophysiology Society guideline 3: A proposal for standard montages to be used in clinical EEG. J Clin Neurophysiol 2016;33:312–316.

10. Epstein, CM. Aliasing in the visual EEG: A potential pitfall of video display technology. Clin Neurophysiol 2003;114:1974–1976.

CHAPTER 3

Rules of localization

One of the main aims of electroencephalogram (EEG) analysis is to solve the inverse problem: localizing the source based on the EEG activity captured on the scalp. This is particularly relevant for epileptiform discharges based on which we attempt to localize the seizure focus in the brain. In this chapter, we will be discussing rules of localization in relation to epileptiform spikes, but the same principles are broadly applicable to other sources and corresponding EEG manifestations (e.g., a tumor giving rise to EEG slow waves).

One must be familiar with three principles to understand the rules of localization: (1) rules of polarity, (2) rules of voltage fields, and (3) montages. Some elements have already been discussed under the volume conduction theory in Chapter 1. Additionally, it should be emphasized that we work with certain assumptions to simplify the process of localization. First, we assume that our solution is a point source single generator such as an equivalent current dipole. The second assumption is that the head is a homogenous volume conductor. Finally, in relation to epileptiform discharges, we usually consider the dipole to be surface-negative, i.e., the negative pole is directed toward the surface (scalp), though in horizontal and tangential dipoles, we will also capture positivity on the scalp.

RULES OF POLARITY

The waveforms we observe on EEGs have either upward or downward deflections relative to the baseline. Polarity is a convention for labeling these deflections. It is always determined in relation to the input 1 and input 2 of the differential amplifier. There are only four simple rules to remember:

1. Input 1 – Input 2 = output signal.
2. If input 1 – input 2 = a negative value, the outcome signal shows an upward deflection (negative deflection). This situation arises if input 1 is relatively more negative than input 2 or input 1 is relatively less positive than input 2.
3. If input 1 – input 2 = a positive value, the outcome signal shows a downward deflection (positive deflection). This situation arises if input 1 is relatively more positive than input 2 or input 1 is relatively less negative than input 2.
4. If input 1 – input 2 = 0, the outcome is a flatline.

These rules are illustrated in Figures 3.1a–f. Figure 3.1a shows a scenario generating an upward deflection (or a negative wave). The input 1 electrode (A) is in the negative voltage field of the dipole and input 2 is in a neutral (0) region. The final outcome (A – B) is negative, hence the deflection is upward. In Figure 3.1b, both inputs are looking at the negative pole, but input 1 is closer to the field maximum, capturing much higher activity than input 2. The final outcome of input 1 – input 2 is still negative, recording a negative spike with a smaller amplitude than in Figure 3.1a. In the third scenario (Figure 3.1c), both electrodes are in the same voltage field (isopotential),

DOI: 10.1201/9781003353713-4

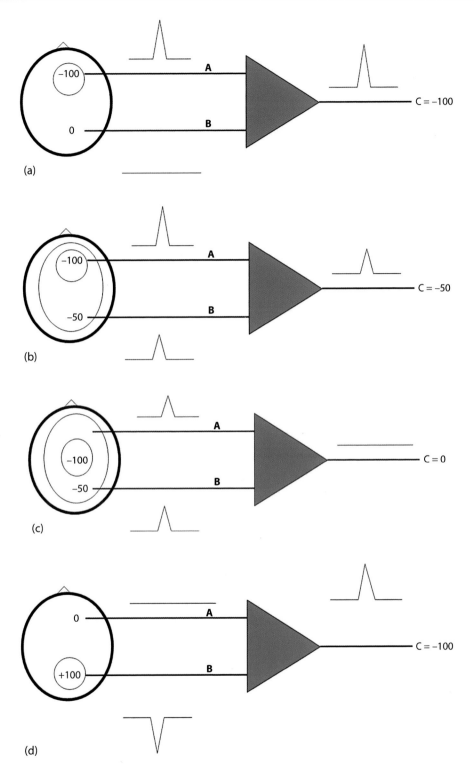

Figure 3.1   Six different scenarios illustrating the rules of polarity. A is input 1 electrode and B is input 2 electrode. C is the output channel. A – B = C. The output is shown here without amplification for simplicity. It should be remembered that output potential is always amplified with the use of amplifiers in EEG recordings. (a) C is a negative value, hence, the deflection is upward. (b) C is a negative value, hence, the deflection is upward. (c) C is equal to 0, hence, there is no deflection. (d) C is a negative value, hence, the deflection is upward. (e) C is a positive value, hence, the deflection is downward. (f) C is a negative value, hence, the deflection is upward. *(Continued)*

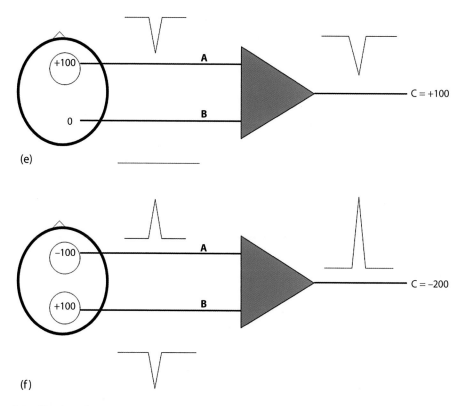

Figure 3.1 *(Continued)*

hence, the final outcome is equal to zero generating a flatline. In Figure 3.1d, input 1 is in a neutral region whereas input 2 is in the voltage field of the positive end of the dipole. This also gives rise to a negative spike as input 1 − input 2 is still a negative value. In the next scenario (Figure 3.1e), input 1 is close to the positive pole whilst input 2 is in a neutral region. Hence, the final outcome is positive, generating a downward deflection. In the final scenario (Figure 3.1f), inputs 1 and 2 are located at the opposite ends of the dipole. The final outcome (A − B) is a negative value generating an upward deflection.

It is important to emphasize here that a flatline does not necessarily mean the absence of activity in the brain. As shown in Figure 3.1c, if both inputs capture equal potentials, the outcome is a flatline. It is the way differential amplifiers work. We never see an EEG signal output with a single input, as differential amplifiers always need two inputs. Even when we use a reference, there are two inputs with the reference being input 2. How can we find out the absolute potential at a point in the brain? We can achieve this by placing the input 2 electrode on a neutral point (as in Figure 3.1a). However, this is not practical as we do not have *a priori* knowledge of the field. Hence, the only option is to use a neutral reference electrode as input 2. In reality, it is not possible to find a location with zero activity, so we aim to find a reference point close to zero. This is the basis of the referential montages we have discussed.

It is not uncommon to see both positive and negative deflections within the same waveform complex. This happens when complex waveforms are captured.

VOLTAGE FIELDS

This section must be read in conjunction with the volume conduction theory and solid angle theory described in Chapter 1. Figure 3.2 shows a current dipole consisting of pyramidal neurons radially oriented within a homogeneous volume conductor. For simplicity, the brain is considered

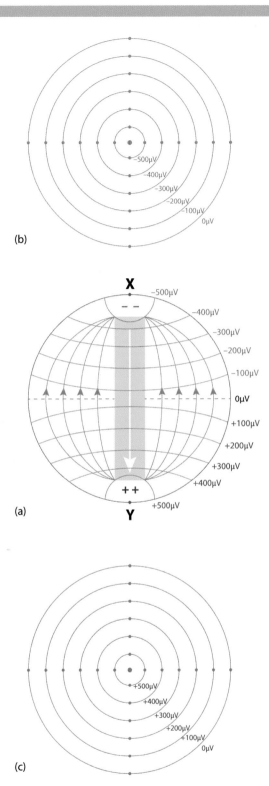

Figure 3.2 Generation of a voltage field by a current dipole. (a) Current flows from "source" to "sink" around the dipole source externally. Voltage fields are generated by combining the points intersecting the current flow with lines drawn at a right angle to each line of current flow. The line that combines spots with the same potential is called an isopotential line. (b) Voltage field map of the negative pole. This represents the bird's-eye view of the pole at X. Each isopotential line is generated by combining multiple spots with equal potentials (represented by blue dots). Each blue dot represents an intersection with the current flow. (c) Voltage field map of the positive pole. This represents the bird's-eye view of the pole at Y.

a spherical volume conductor here. Current flows extracellularly from "source" to "sink" through the volume conductor. The current density gradually falls as it moves further away from the dipole source. Along with that, a voltage field develops. The highest potential is close to the epicenter of the dipole and the voltage drops off as the distance increases from the pole as described by Gloor.[1] We can combine the spots with similar potentials (isopotential lines) and the result is an isopotential field map, as shown in Figure 3.2b & c. What we measure on the scalp is also determined by the solid angle subtended. In the most simplistic model, with a radial dipole, the electrode placed right on top of the pole will record the maximum potential. The voltage gradually decreases with increasing electrode distances, simulating the isopotential maps shown in Figure 3.2b & c and Figure 1.3 in Chapter 1. In a radial dipole, as shown in the Figure 1.3, the negative voltage field will be captured on the scalp electrodes. The positive voltage field cannot be captured in real life, though it exists, as there is no way to place electrodes over that pole (base of the skull). In the case of horizontal and oblique dipoles (Chapter 1, Figures 1.4 and 1.5), isopotential maps for both positive and negative potentials can be plotted over the scalp. All electrodes placed at different locations but within the same isopotential field will subtend the same solid angle and record the same voltage.

MONTAGES

The rules of localization must be discussed in relation to montages as it is how we read EEGs in routine practice. What is a montage? The two electrodes providing inputs to a single amplifier form an "electrode derivation."[2] For example, if inputs 1 and 2 are from F7 and T3 electrodes, the electrode derivation is F7–T3. When electrode derivations are linked in a logical manner to enhance the visual display, the combined arrangement is referred to as a "montage."[2] There are many different ways derivations can be combined to form montages. The bipolar and the referential montages are the fundamental groups. The American Clinical Neurophysiology Society recommends the use of both bipolar and referential montages in EEG reading and interpretation.[3]

Localization rules with bipolar montages

Bipolar montages are created like chains with input 2 of one derivation becoming the input 1 of the next derivation except for the two electrodes at the beginning and the end. The connections can be along the longitudinal axis (longitudinal bipolar montage) or transverse axis (transverse bipolar montage). Along these two axes are many ways to connect adjoining electrodes to generate the "chains." However the electrodes are joined, the localizing rules for the bipolar montages are the same. In fact, this is a very clever montage arrangement to make abnormalities stand out to catch the attention of the reader; electroencephalographers often use a bipolar montage to screen the EEG first. Bipolar montages are particularly useful to discover low-amplitude potentials with a narrow field buried in a background of high-amplitude potentials of wide special distribution due to phase cancellation of the background activity. For the same reason, if the potential of interest has a wide spatial distribution, it will not stand out for easy identification on a bipolar montage.

The key feature to look for in the visual analysis of the bipolar montage is phase reversal. Phase refers to the deflection of the EEG waveform in a particular direction. On a bipolar montage, phase reversal is reflected by waveform deflections in two or more channels in opposite directions. If the deflections are toward a particular channel or electrode, it is called a negative phase reversal. A positive phase reversal is characterized by waveforms moving away from a channel or electrode. It is important to emphasize that phase reversal is not a biological phenomenon. It is a visual phenomenon created by the bipolar montage due to the way electrodes are connected in the chain. For that reason, this phenomenon is also called "instrumental phase reversal." The center of the phase reversal, both negative and positive, indicates where the maximum potential is (Figures 3.3 and 3.4).

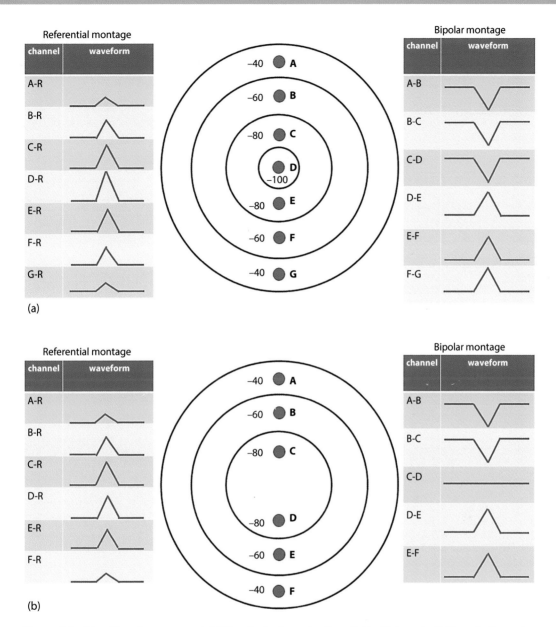

Figure 3.3 **Negative phase reversal.** (a) Negatively charged voltage field with isopotential lines. In the center of the field, the maximum voltage is 100 μV and the values get lower as you move away from the epicenter to the periphery. A–G are electrodes placed in this field. Please note the voltage values are only arbitrary values to explain the concept. **Bipolar montage:** The output of each channel is equal to input 1 – input 2. Negative phase reversal occurs at D electrode, which has the maximum voltage. **Referential montage:** Input 2 is a reference electrode with zero potential. Hence the output of each channel in this montage is equal to the absolute potential of each input 1 electrode. (b) Another presentation of negative phase reversal. Electrodes C and D are isopotential, generating a flatline on bipolar montage. Negative phase reversal occurs on either side of the flatline. In this situation, the intervening channel with phase cancellation (C–D flatline) represents the field maximum. The referential montage shows this clearly.

In radial dipoles, the source is underneath the amplitude maxima, as discussed in Chapter 1 (Figure 1.3). The center of phase reversal could also be the focus of minimum potential as illustrated in Figure 3.5. This rather theoretical situation can arise with two adjacent dipoles when the negative (or positive) ends of each dipole are captured on the scalp with electrodes aligned across both fields, as shown in Figure 3.5.

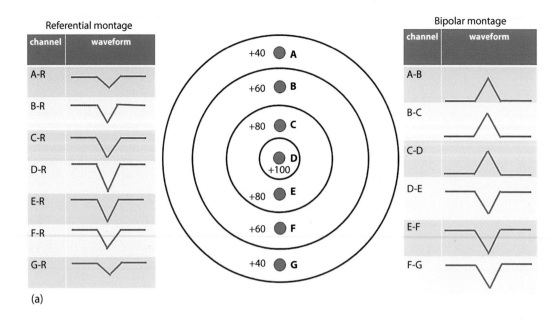

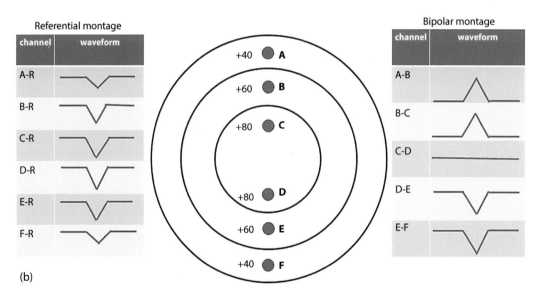

Figure 3.4 Positive phase reversal. (a) Positively charged voltage field with isopotential lines. The electrode placement and interpretation are similar to Figure 3.3a. **Bipolar montage:** Positive phase reversal is seen at the D electrode, which has the maximum potential. **Referential montage:** The explanation is similar to Figure 3.3a. (b) Positive phase reversal with phase cancellation in the intervening channel. C and D electrodes are isopotential, generating a flatline on the bipolar montage and positive phase reversal occurs on either side. The referential montage reflects the voltage field with maxima at C and D electrodes.

The presence of phase reversal does not necessarily indicate pathological activity. Physiological waveforms such as vertex waves in sleep also demonstrate phase reversal. It is simply a way of demonstrating the locations of the maximum (or minimum) potential of a field.

If the generator is an oblique or a horizontal dipole, both positive and negative phase reversals can be observed simultaneously. This phenomenon is called a double phase reversal (Figure 3.6). As discussed in Chapter 1, in a horizontal dipole, the source is underneath the minimum field

Referential montage

channel	waveform
A-R	
B-R	
C-R	
D-R	
E-R	
F-R	
G-R	

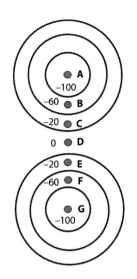

Bipolar montage

channel	waveform
A-B	
B-C	
C-D	
D-E	
E-F	
F-G	

Figure 3.5 Phase reversal at the point of minimum potential. Voltage fields (both negative) of two adjacent dipoles are shown here. Electrodes are placed across both fields. **Bipolar montage:** Note positive phase reversal at electrode D, which has the lowest potential of zero. Referential montage confirms the minimum potential of zero at D.

Referential montage

channel	waveform
A-R	
B-R	
C-R	
D-R	
E-R	
F-R	
G-R	
H-R	
I-R	
J-R	
K-R	

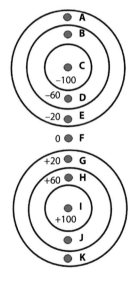

Bipolar montage

channel	waveform
A-B	
B-C	
C-D	
D-E	
E-F	
F-G	
G-H	
H-I	
I-J	
J-K	

Figure 3.6 Double phase reversal due to a horizontal dipole. Both negative and positive ends and respective voltage fields of the dipole are captured on the scalp. Electrodes are placed across both the voltage fields. **Bipolar montage:** Note negative phase reversal at C (electrode with the maximum negative potential) and positive phase reversal at I (electrode with the maximum positive potential). As both positive and negative phase reversals are captured synchronously, this phenomenon is called double phase reversal. **Referential montage:** Potentials at each electrode demonstrate the voltage field with the negative maximum at C and positive maximum at I.

potential (Figure 1.4), located in the midpoint between positive and negative phase reversals. However, in an oblique dipole, the field minimum is shifted away from the source, as shown in Chapter 1 (Figure 1.5).

What will happen if the field maxima are located at the extreme end of the electrode chain or beyond? In such a case, phase reversal does not occur as there is no electrode to record the activity

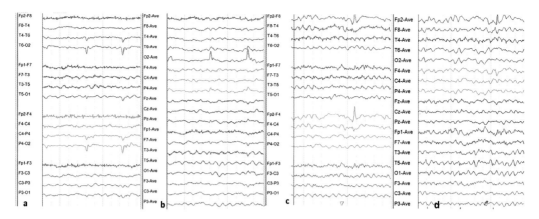

Figure 3.7   End-of-chain phenomenon at the occipital and frontal ends of the chain. (a) Sharp waves in the right occipital region (T6O2, P4O2) show no phase reversal in the longitudinal bipolar montage. (b) Referential montage confirms that the voltage maximum is at O2. As it is the last posterior electrode in the chain, there is no way to demonstrate phase reversal. (c) Sharp waves in the right frontal region (Fp2F8, Fp2F4) show no phase reversal in the longitudinal bipolar montage. (d) Referential montage confirms that the voltage maximum is at Fp2. As it is the last anterior electrode in the chain, there is no way to demonstrate phase reversal.

beyond the point of maxima. Hence, all deflections will be in one direction. This is identified as the "end-of-chain phenomenon" (Figure 3.7).

Two bipolar montages in longitudinal and transverse axes should be applied for more precise localization. Having discussed those phenomena, the rules of localization based on the bipolar montage can be summarized as follows:

1. When phase reversal is evident, the maximum or minimum activity is located at the electrode or electrodes around which the phase reversal occurs.

2. When there is no phase reversal, the minimum and maximum activity are located at either end of the chain.

3. The absence of any deflection in a given channel indicates that the two inputs have the same potential.

Localization rules with referential montages

In a referential montage, input 2 is common across all derivations whereas the individual electrodes form input 1 in each derivation. Hence, by nature of this arrangement, we are not looking for phase reversals. In fact, the main aim of a referential montage is to study the "absolute voltage" at each individual electrode and the key component of interest is the amplitude of waveforms. To achieve this target, the reference electrode has to be neutral. In reality, it is nearly impossible to find an electrode with zero activity, hence, the aim would be to select a reference electrode with no involvement in the electrical field of interest and least susceptible to artifacts. The main challenge for the electroencephalographer is reference contamination, and rational judgment is needed to select the appropriate reference in each individual case. There is no single ideal reference that suits all scenarios.

In source localization and studying voltage fields with referential montages, the key component of interest is amplitude. Referential montages are also useful to study the morphology of the waveforms, asymmetries, and phase relations.[4,5]

The rules of localization based on the referential montage can be summarized as follows:

1. If there is no phase reversal (all deflections pointing in the same direction), the reference electrode is located at the minimum or maximum of the field.

2. If an appropriate reference with minimum or no involvement in the field is chosen and no phase reversal occurs, the electrode (input 1) recording the highest amplitude is likely to be over the source, provided the point generator is radial in orientation.

3. If the reference is in the field maximum and no phase reversal occurs, the electrode (input 1) recording the highest amplitude is likely to be at the minimum point of the voltage field.

4. If the reference is in the field maximum and no phase reversal occurs, the electrode (input 1) recording the lowest amplitude is likely to be closer to the maximum point of the voltage field. If any channel shows no deflection, the input 1 electrode of that channel is likely to be at the maximum point of the voltage field.

5. If there is a phase reversal, the reference is neither the minimum nor the maximum. For example, in the case of a voltage field of a surface-negative epileptiform spike, the channels with electrodes at input 1 with a higher voltage than the reference will record an upward deflection, while those channels with input electrodes at a lower voltage will record a downward deflection, resulting in a phase reversal. In practical terms, this situation represents a poor choice of the reference electrode.

6. If an appropriate reference with minimum or no involvement in the field is chosen and phase reversal occurs, the source is likely to be a horizontal or an oblique dipole (Figure 3.6).

PITFALLS AND LIMITATIONS OF LOCALIZATION

A beginner might think that the channel with the highest amplitude is always the focus of maximum activity. It is important to remember this rule is not applicable in bipolar montages, as the output represents the difference between the two inputs. In a bipolar montage, one must always look for phase reversals rather than amplitude. If there is no phase reversal, the next step is to look for the "end-of-chain phenomenon." A likely cause of confusion with the bipolar montage is a potential with a wide field. Due to in-phase cancellations, the phase reversal may not be obvious, or it may be completely missed as the difference between adjacent electrodes is so small.

The main challenge in the use of the referential montage is "reference contamination," when the reference electrode happens to be within the voltage field. As a result, spurious phase reversals and pseudo-dipoles may be generated that can be misinterpreted as true phenomena by an inexperienced reader (Figure 3.8).[5,6] In-phase cancellation occurs with the referential montage as well.

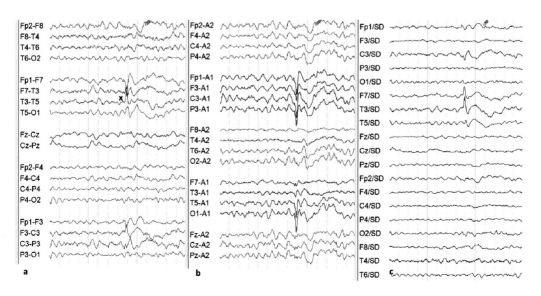

Figure 3.8 Reference contamination. (a) In this longitudinal bipolar montage, negative phase reversal of the sharp wave at T3 suggests that it has the maximum negative potential. (b) Ear reference montage of the same EEG. Unusual positive deflection is seen in multiple channels. This is because the reference electrode A1 is in the voltage field of the sharp wave, hence, the reference is "contaminated." T3 is expected to show the maximum amplitude in a referential montage, but here T3A1 generates a small positive deflection. As A1 has a higher negative potential than T3, the output is a downward deflection. As the difference is small, the deflection has a small amplitude. (c) Source derivation montage confirms T3 voltage and amplitude maxima.

The degree of cancellation depends on the distance between the reference and the input 1 electrode with shorter distances resulting in increasing in-phase cancellations. Hence, if the reference is close to the source, there will be excessive attenuation close to the source resulting in mislocalization.

Paradoxical lateralization occurs when the source is erroneously lateralized to the contralateral hemisphere on the EEG. This phenomenon tends to occur with midline and parasagittal foci. If the dipole is obliquely oriented, the electrodes over the opposite hemisphere will have the best "look" at the source and record the maximum activity in keeping with the solid angle theory.[7] This pitfall should be borne in mind when interpreting sources located in the midline, particularly on the mesial surface (see Chapter 9, Figure 9.3, for an example).

As a reminder, the aforementioned rules are based on the premise that the source is a single generator located within a homogeneous volume conductor. However, in real life, the situation is different. There are several anatomic variants of source configuration such as multiple microfoci, double dipoles, and quadrupoles.[6] Furthermore, different tissue layers between the source and the recording electrode have variable conductivities and, as a result, the scalp EEG maxima can be further away from the generator.[8]

References

1. Gloor, P. Neuronal generators and the problem of localization in electroencephalography: Application of volume conductor theory to electroencephalography. J Clin Neurophysiol 1985;2:327–354.

2. Knott, JR. Further thoughts on polarity, montages, and localization. J Clin Neurophysiol 1985;2:63–75.

3. Acharya, JN, Hani, AJ, Thirumala, PD, Tsuchida, TN. American Clinical Neurophysiology Society guideline 3: A proposal for standard montages to be used in clinical EEG. J Clin Neurophysiol 2016;33:312–316.

4. Cooper, R. An ambiguity of bipolar recording. Electroencephalogr Clin Neurophysiol 1959;11:819–820.

5. Seneviratne, U. Rational manipulation of digital EEG: Pearls and pitfalls. J Clin Neurophysiol 2014;31:507–516.

6. Jayakar, P, Duchowny, M, Resnick, TJ, Alvarez, LA. Localization of seizure foci: Pitfalls and caveats. J Clin Neurophysiol 1991;8:414–431.

7. Adelman, S, Lueders, H, Dinner, DS, Lesser, RP. Paradoxical lateralization of parasagittal sharp waves in a patient with epilepsia partialis continua. Epilepsia 1982;23:291–295.

8. Perrin, F, Bertrand, O, Giard, MH, Pernier, J. Precautions in topographic mapping and in evoked potential map reading. J Clin Neurophysiol 1990;7:498–506.

Normal EEG

CHAPTER 4

Visual analysis of EEG
A systematic approach

The electroencephalogram (EEG) should be approached akin to an anatomical dissection of the body. The reader must review each epoch and break it down into several components for a systematic analysis. Finally, those elements must be resynthesized epoch by epoch for the entire recording in a meaningful way for interpretation. This chapter is dedicated to "EEG anatomy," i.e., the description of multiple components of an EEG. The subsequent chapters describe how to resynthesize those components for the final interpretation.

EEG can be visualized as a graph plotted in two domains: spatial distribution (*y*-axis) and temporal distribution (*x*-axis). All EEG characteristics can be dissected and analyzed along these axes.

Before studying the individual EEG characteristics, the reader must ask some preliminary questions:

1. What is the age of the subject? Age is a critical factor to interpret the findings after the initial "dissection." EEG characteristics change as the brain matures. Some hypersynchronous EEG activity such as hypnogogic hypersynchrony is a normal finding in children. Some slow activities (e.g., temporal theta) are considered normal in the elderly. Certain normal variants are seen in particular age groups (e.g., posterior slow wave of youth).

2. What is the level of alertness/vigilance state of the subject? Similarly, the level of alertness, both physiological (awake versus sleep) and pathological (stupor, coma), will influence how we interpret certain EEG features (e.g., alpha rhythm versus alpha coma). The identification of wakefulness and sleep will be discussed in the next chapter.

3. What is the EEG montage on display? The importance of montages has been discussed in a previous chapter. What we see in the epoch depends on the montage. Before analyzing EEG features, the reader must know which montage is on display and change it if necessary.

4. Were any activation procedures conducted during the recording?

   Hyperventilation and photic stimulation are carried out routinely as activation procedures during EEG recording. It is important to note in a given epoch whether an activation procedure was conducted in order to determine the significance of EEG changes. For example, generalized delta slowing during hyperventilation is a normal finding. However, the same feature may indicate encephalopathy if occurs spontaneously.

THE EEG ANATOMY

Morphology

Waveforms are fundamental building blocks of the EEG. Each waveform has an amplitude, duration, and shape. The characteristic shapes are referred to as morphology. Sharp waves and spikes are narrow transients with a pointed peak. Mu rhythm consists of arch-like (arciform) waves. Slow waves

DOI: 10.1201/9781003353713-6

are dome-shaped. Zeta waves have a Z-like configuration. The concept of "phase" is closely linked with morphology and determined by the number of instances the waveform crosses the baseline. The number of phases is equal to the number of baseline crossings + 1. For example, if a waveform crosses the baseline two times, it has three phases.

Symmetry

The EEG characteristics such as amplitude, frequency, rhythmicity, and abundance should be approximately symmetrical between homologous brain regions. If there is an asymmetry, as a general rule, the side with "less/lower" activity is abnormal. Asymmetry in amplitude and frequency are particularly important. On a referential montage, peak-to-trough amplitude difference of <50% or frequency difference of 0.5–1 Hz is considered mild asymmetry whereas marked asymmetry is defined as amplitude difference of ≥50% or frequency difference of >1 Hz.

Frequency

Waveforms spread along a time domain and, hence, have an integral frequency. The scalp EEG consists of a mix of several frequency bands. The frequency is measured in terms of cycles per second (Hertz). For example, if you find three cycles (or waveforms) within a time span of 1 second, the frequency is 3 Hz. Most routinely studied frequencies are within the bandwidth of 0.5 to 70 Hz. The frequency bands found in the scalp EEG are[1]:

- Infraslow: <0.1 Hz
- Delta: 0.1–<4 Hz
- Theta: 4–<8 Hz
- Alpha: 8–13 Hz
- Beta: >13–30 Hz
- Gamma: >30–80 Hz
- High frequency oscillations:
  - High gamma: 80–150 Hz
  - Ripples: 80–250 Hz
  - Fast ripples: 250–500 Hz

The EEG reader should be very cautious in the interpretation of very slow frequencies as those are more likely to be artifacts or extracerebral in origin. True infraslow activity is considered helpful in localizing the seizure onset zone. Similarly, pathological high frequency oscillations are a marker of the seizure onset zone.[2]

Amplitude

The amplitude is usually measured from baseline to peak or peak to trough. Amplitude should never be measured in a bipolar montage as phase cancellation leads to erroneous results. In the scalp EEG, the amplitude of the waveforms usually ranges from 20 to 100 microvolts. In contrast, amplitudes recorded in electrocorticography are in the range of 500 to 1,500 microvolts. Marked asymmetry refers to a 50% or more difference in peak-to-trough voltage or a >1 Hz difference in frequency of EEG activities including the posterior dominant rhythm between the hemispheres.[1] Reduced amplitude over a hemisphere may be due to an increased distance between the cerebral cortex and the electrode (e.g., subdural hematoma) or some dysfunction of the hemisphere (e.g., hypoperfusion). More commonly, the reduced amplitude is due to technical factors such as reduced interelectrode distance or a salt bridge. On the contrary, a higher amplitude over a region can be the result of a defect in the skull (breach rhythm) (Figure 4.1). Other characteristics of the breach rhythm are admixed fast components and sharply contoured mu-like activity.[3] Some individuals

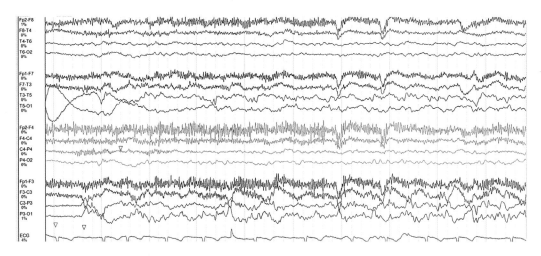

Figure 4.1   Breach rhythm over the left posterior head region. Note the higher amplitude of waveforms compared with homologous right-sided channels with a mixture of fast and slow rhythms.

have amplitudes of <20 microvolts across all the electrodes (low-voltage EEG), which is a normal variant.[1] EEG amplitudes of <10 microvolts are referred to as suppression observed in the setting of encephalopathy, particularly due to hypoxia, ischemia, and certain medications.

Rhythms

Rhythm refers to an EEG activity consisting of waveforms of equal duration. When those waveforms recur at the same frequency, the activity is identified as rhythmic. When we describe rhythmicity, the key element is the duration of the waveform, and hence frequency. Regularity refers to the morphology of the EEG waveform. When the waveforms of identical morphology recur, those are called regular (monomorphic). The opposite is irregular (polymorphic) activity. Based on the waveform duration and morphology, we can see three possible combinations: rhythmic regular activity, rhythmic irregular activity, and arrhythmic irregular activity (Figure 4.2a–c).

Reactivity

Reactivity refers to clear and reproducible changes in EEG activity in its frequency, amplitude, or morphology in response to sensory stimuli.[1] It is a key feature of the alpha rhythm that will be discussed in the next chapter. EEG reactivity is considered a good prognostic sign in comatose patients.

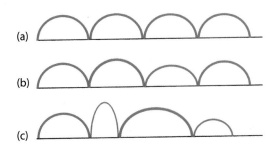

Figure 4.2   Three types of rhythmic activity. (a) Regular, rhythmic; (b) Irregular, rhythmic; (c) Irregular, arrhythmic.

Synchrony

Synchrony is an EEG characteristic related to the time domain. When a certain type of EEG activity occurs in two brain regions in the same hemisphere or opposite hemispheres simultaneously, it is identified as synchrony. Bilateral synchrony or bisynchrony is used to identify activities emerging at the same time in homologous brain regions. The best-known example of bisynchrony is the generalized spike-wave activity in idiopathic generalized epilepsies.

Spatial distribution

As discussed in Chapter 3, EEG activity has a field that determines spatial distribution. When the EEG activity is bilateral and synchronous, as in the case of generalized spike-wave discharges, it is identified as generalized. The term "diffuse" is used in a relatively less restrictive sense to describe EEG activities spread over large areas bilaterally. "Focal" refers to a small area of the brain whereas "regional" indicates the involvement of a particular lobe (e.g., frontal, temporal). "Multifocal" means three or more spatially separated multiple areas (foci) and "multiregional" refers to the involvement of three or more lobes. Any activity spread across an entire hemisphere is identified as lateralized activity.[1]

Complexes, transients, bursts, and paroxysms

EEG waveforms appear in isolation or combination. When two or more waveforms combine to form a characteristic morphology, which occurs consistently distinguishable from the background, it is called a complex. The spike-wave complex is a good example. A transient is any single waveform or a complex that stands out from the background. Transients can be physiological or pathological (e.g., sleep transient versus epileptiform sharp waves). Bursts are characterized by a sequence of waveforms having a minimum of four phases emerging from the background with an abrupt onset and offset lasting >0.5 seconds. Bursts can be normal or abnormal. Paroxysms are EEG waveforms that suddenly emerge from the background, reach the peak rapidly, are sustained, and then terminate abruptly. This term is generally reserved for epileptiform and seizure patterns.[1] Contrary to bursts, the number of phases and duration are not predefined in paroxysms.

Prevalence of EEG activity

When an EEG abnormality is detected, it is important to express how prevalent the abnormality is within the recording. This can be expressed at the epoch level as well as record level and should be specified as such. If the activity occupies ≥90% of the record/epoch, it is identified as a continuous activity (e.g., continuous generalized slowing). Less than 90% prevalence is called intermittent. In critical care EEG, intermittent abnormalities or activities are subdivided into abundant (EEG activity occupies 50–89% of epoch/record), frequent (10–49%), occasional (1–9%), and rare (<1%).[4]

Periodicity

In some situations, EEG complexes and waveforms tend to recur at regular intervals. This phenomenon is referred to as periodicity, which is particularly relevant in critical care EEG. Periodic lateralized discharges and periodic generalized discharges are good examples in the context of critical care EEG. This will be discussed in more detail in Chapter 15. Focal epilepsy due to focal cortical dysplasia is another condition where periodic epileptiform discharges are witnessed. The American Clinical Neurophysiology Society (ACNS) defines periodic as "repetition of a waveform with relatively uniform morphology and duration with a quantifiable inter-discharge interval between consecutive waveforms and recurrence of the waveform at nearly regular intervals."[4] It should be noted that the intervals between complexes are allowed to be "nearly regular," which means periods (intervals) can vary by <50% in the sequential pair of cycles in >50% pairs of the record.[4] Furthermore, the recurring activity should last at least six cycles to qualify as a periodic pattern. For example, if the complexes recur at a frequency of 1 Hz, it should continue for at least 6 seconds to meet the criteria of a periodic pattern (Figure 4.3).[4]

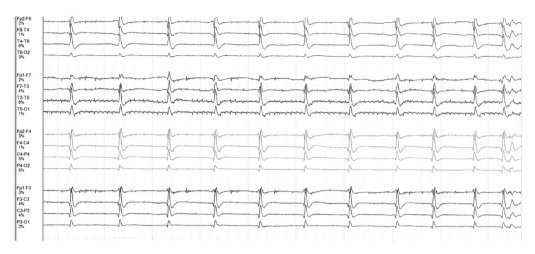

Figure 4.3 Periodicity. Note the discharges recure at 1 Hz frequency persisting for >6 seconds, fulfilling the criteria for a periodic pattern.

ESSENTIAL STEPS IN READING THE EEG

There is no hard-and-fast rule as to how one should study an EEG. One's approach is usually defined by experience and refined by practice. The steps given here are only a guide for the beginner. How to read a critical care EEG is described in Chapter 18. The key to reading any EEG is paying attention to the details. There must be an explanation for every change you see on the EEG record. Reading the EEG is an art combined with the science of neurophysiology and enhanced by the skill of pattern recognition.

1. Study the background information as detailed at the beginning of this chapter. Be guided by those data but not biased. Never try to find changes on the EEG to fit the clinical picture or the question raised in the request.

2. Open the EEG and study the settings. Pay attention to the filters, sensitivity, timebase, and montages. Be familiar with the EEG software used in your laboratory.

3. Look for a posterior dominant rhythm. If the patient is awake and responsive, the technologist will usually check reactivity at the beginning of the recording.

4. Go through the EEG page (epoch) by page. Each page can be 10, 20, or 30 seconds depending on the lab. Do not hesitate to change the timebase when necessary. When there is an abnormality such as an evolving rhythm, scrolling the EEG second by second is more useful.

5. Note the state of vigilance in each epoch.

6. Study the general background in each epoch. Dissect the EEG anatomy of the background as detailed in this chapter.

7. Look for any changes from the normal background (of the vigilance state). Any deviation from the normal background activity must be a normal variant, epileptiform abnormality, non-epileptiform abnormality, or an artifact. Once you have completed reading this book, you will know how to recognize changes belonging to those four categories.

8. Study the EEG anatomy and make note of all deviations from the normal background.

9. Get used to a single montage as the "screening" montage. My recommendation is the longitudinal bipolar montage. Whenever you see a deviation from the normal background, apply other montages (such as a referential montage or a transverse montage) to study that change in more detail. Do not hesitate to change other settings in a rational way for a more detailed analysis of the EEG alteration, as discussed in Chapter 2.

10. If the entire EEG looks normal on the screening montage, study it again from the beginning at least one more time, using a referential montage to make sure subtle abnormalities have not been missed.

11. Do not forget the electrocardiograph (ECG) channel. You can train your eye to study the ECG with EEG signals in each epoch. If it is difficult, study the ECG channel separately after completing the EEG reading.

12. Pay particular attention to the four blind spots (described in Chapter 18).

13. Pay attention to the annotations made by the technologist.

14. Study the synchronous video for clinical-EEG correlation. Modern EEG machines are almost always equipped with video recording. Viewing the video at the beginning is also recommended to have a good understanding of the state of the patient and the environment.

15. Do not rush. Spend sufficient time to study the EEG. If there is any doubt, go through the EEG again and again. Do not hesitate to get opinions from colleagues.

16. Finally, when you are satisfied, prepare to generate the report. Classify the abnormalities, summarize the findings, and interpret the findings in the final report.

ESSENTIAL COMPONENTS OF AN EEG REPORT

The EEG report is the final product of the EEG reading. It is the channel of communication between the electroencephalographer and the clinician who requested the study. Hence, it is important to pay close attention to the report. It should be objective, clear, and useful to the clinician. Ambiguities at all levels should be avoided. The ACNS has published guidelines on EEG reporting.[5] Essential components of an EEG report are summarized here.

Identification details

Demographic and identification details of the patient including the hospital identification number are contained on top of the report. Details of the hospital or EEG lab and contact information are often included. Some EEG labs may include the name of the referring doctor.

Technical details

This is an integral part of any EEG report. It should contain the type of EEG (routine, ambulatory, short-term video, sleep-deprived, etc.) as well as the date and time of the recording. The electrode setup, whether 10–20 system or any other variation, should be described. It is very important to include the activation procedures such as hyperventilation and photic stimulation used. Furthermore, the setting of the EEG recording (e.g., in the intensive care unit under sedation of an intubated patient) should be mentioned. If the patient was under sedation at the time of EEG recording, those medication details are very relevant to the EEG reader and should be noted in the report.

History

This section contains clinical details that help the electroencephalographer interpret the findings correctly. The indication for EEG should be explicit. The current clinical problem, relevant history, relevant family history, current medications, and relevant investigations including previous EEGs are essential. However, the information presented here should be concise.

State of consciousness

The level of vigilance can vary during the recording and all states observed should be noted here. It is usually very brief: awake, drowsy, asleep, or altered conscious state.

EEG description

This section summarizes what you found in your analysis of the EEG. The description usually starts with statements on the posterior dominant rhythm followed by the general (nondominant) background. All descriptions here should be objective. All abnormalities need to be described with sufficient details as described in this chapter. It is good practice to include normal variants and significant artifacts. Outcomes of activation procedures, whether normal or abnormal, should be noted. It is important to note state changes including sleep stages. It may be relevant to mention some important negatives, such as the absence of epileptiform discharges.

Video recording is a routine practice now with any EEG recording. Whenever relevant events are observed, the semiology should be described after viewing the video. The description should include the time of onset as well as offset.

Finally, one must not forget to describe the findings of the single-channel ECG. If any other polygraphy channels (such as pulse oximetry or electromyography) were used in selected patients, those findings should be noted.

EEG classification

This is a summary of the outcome expressed with a single word: normal or abnormal. If the EEG is abnormal, it is good practice to grade the degree of abnormality. There is no universally accepted system. One proposed classification has three grades of abnormality: abnormal I, II, and III.[6] If there are significant abnormalities, it would be useful to list a summary of abnormalities. Example:

Abnormal III

1. Intermittent sharp waves – left temporal
2. Intermittent slow – left temporal
3. Posterior dominant background – slow

Impression and clinical correlation

This is the final section of the EEG report, and it needs good attention as this is the most relevant section to the referring doctor. The summary of EEG findings is synthesized into a clinically relevant message here. It should be simple enough so that someone without any background EEG knowledge should be able to understand the message. EEG is a test, but not a consult. Hence, an EEG report is not a place to provide direct advice on patient management such as starting or ceasing antiseizure medications. It may be appropriate to provide some limited guidance such as suggestions to repeat the EEG.

References

1. Kane, N, Acharya, J, Benickzy, S, et al. A revised glossary of terms most commonly used by clinical electroencephalographers and updated proposal for the report format of the EEG findings. Revision 2017. Clin Neurophysiol Pract 2017;2:170–185.

2. Lee, S, Issa, NP, Rose, S, et al. DC shifts, high frequency oscillations, ripples and fast ripples in relation to the seizure onset zone. Seizure 2020;77:52–58.

3. Cobb, WA, Guiloff, RJ, Cast, J. Breach rhythm: The EEG related to skull defects. Electroencephalogr Clin Neurophysiol 1979;47:251–271.

4. Hirsch, LJ, LaRoche, SM, Gaspard, N, et al. American Clinical Neurophysiology Society's Standardized Critical Care EEG Terminology: 2012 version. J Clin Neurophysiol 2013;30:1–27.

5. Tatum, WO, Olga, S, Ochoa, JG, et al. American Clinical Neurophysiology Society Guideline 7: Guidelines for EEG reporting. J Clin Neurophysiol 2016;33:328–332.

6. Luders, H, Noachtar, S. Atlas and Classification of Electroencephalography. Philadelphia: W.B. Saunders, 2000.

CHAPTER 5

Normal EEG in adults

To understand the abnormal electroencephalogram (EEG) well, the reader should first master the features of normal EEG and its variants. This chapter describes characteristics of normal EEG in wakefulness and sleep, whilst Chapter 8 is dedicated to normal EEG variants. An important question to ask when reading an EEG is, "What is the state of vigilance of the subject?" In any normal EEG, the state can be either wakefulness or sleep. Drowsiness, a term often used in EEG reports, is in fact, part of sleep. Specific EEG rhythms, eye movements, sleep transients, and muscle artifacts provide useful clues to distinguish between wakefulness and sleep.

NORMAL EEG IN WAKEFULNESS

The presence of eye blinks, horizontal eye movements, and muscle artifacts indicates wakefulness. However, for a systematic study of the awake EEG, one must break it down into several components, such as frequency of rhythms, amplitude, spatial distribution, and reactivity.

Alpha rhythm

Alpha rhythm is the hallmark of wakefulness. It is characterized by 8–13 Hz of activity symmetrically distributed over the posterior head regions with occipital maxima and accompanied by reactivity (Figure 5.1). It is also called posterior dominant rhythm (PDR), as in some situations the frequency may be below the alpha range.

The frequency of PDR increases with brain maturation to reach the alpha frequency band. It is approximately 4 Hz at 4 months of age and reaches 8 Hz at 3 years. At the age of 9 years, the majority have an alpha rhythm of 9 Hz.[1] Although a mild reduction in alpha frequency may be seen in the elderly, no significant correlation between PDR alpha frequency and age has been found in healthy adults.[2] Slow PDR (<8 Hz) in the elderly is abnormal and usually due to cerebrovascular disease or neurodegenerative conditions including dementia. In any age group, the slowing of PDR is one of the earliest signs of encephalopathy. As detailed in the previous chapter, a frequency difference of >1 Hz between the hemispheres is considered abnormal. The mean frequency of alpha rhythm can vary by 0.5 Hz within an individual recording. In the first 0.5–1 second immediately after eye closure, a transient increase of the frequency up to 3 Hz above the mean can be observed.[3] This phenomenon is known as "alpha squeak."

The amplitude of the alpha rhythm tends to be higher in children compared with adults. One study found the average amplitude (T5-O1 derivation) to be 50–60 microvolts in children aged 3–15 years. Approximately 10% of the healthy population demonstrates an alpha rhythm of low-amplitude <20 microvolts (low-voltage or "flat" EEG) (Figure 5.2).[4] Hyperventilation is a useful activation procedure to increase the amplitude to make it more discernible in those cases. The right hemisphere tends to demonstrate a higher amplitude than the left. Consistent amplitude asymmetries of >50% should be considered abnormal, as discussed in the previous chapter (Figure 5.3).

DOI: 10.1201/9781003353713-7

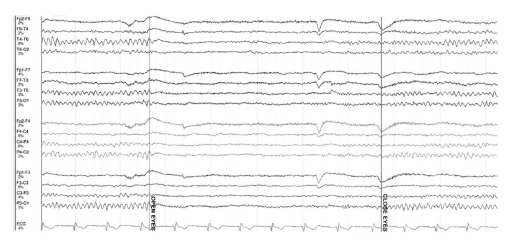

Figure 5.1   Posterior dominant alpha rhythm. Note the reactivity – attenuation with eye opening and amplitude increases with eye closure.

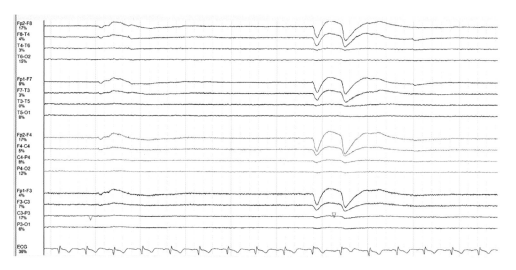

Figure 5.2   Normal EEG with low amplitude. The sensitivity of this epoch is set at 20 μV/mm. Note the "flat" lines with no visible brain activity of >20 μV.

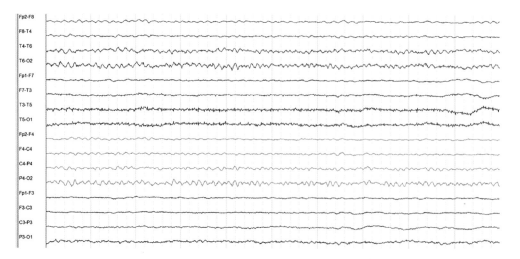

Figure 5.3   Asymmetrical alpha. Note attenuation of all EEG activities, including posterior dominant rhythm over the left hemisphere, due to a subdural hemorrhage on the left.

The waveforms of alpha rhythm are sinusoidal, dome-shaped, or sometimes sharply contoured. Typically, it is maximal over the posterior head regions and occasionally the spatial distribution is parietal, central, posterior temporal, or more widespread.

Reactivity to stimuli is a key feature of the normal alpha rhythm. The alpha rhythm is best demonstrated when the eyes are closed with both physical and mental relaxation. It is blocked or attenuated in amplitude with eye-opening (reactivity) (Figure 5.1). Other sensory stimuli and cognitive activities may also elicit reactivity. Loss of reactivity in one hemisphere, known as the Bancaud phenomenon, suggests an underlying structural abnormality or dysfunction (Figure 5.4a & b).[5] The alpha rhythm usually disappears during drowsiness, but may paradoxically appear with eye-opening (paradoxical alpha) (Figure 5.5).

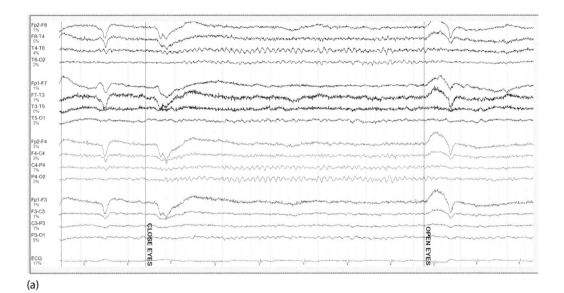

(a)

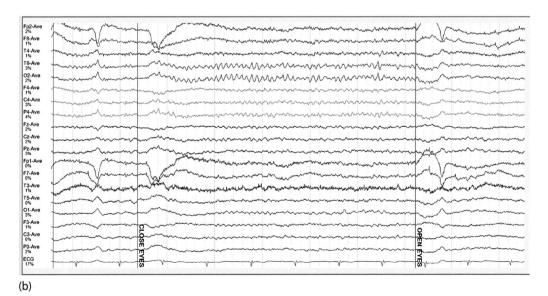

(b)

Figure 5.4   Bancaud phenomenon. Note the lack of alpha reactivity with eye opening on the left on longitudinal bipolar montage (a) and average reference montage (b). The MRI brain scan shows a large area of infarction involving the left cerebral hemisphere.

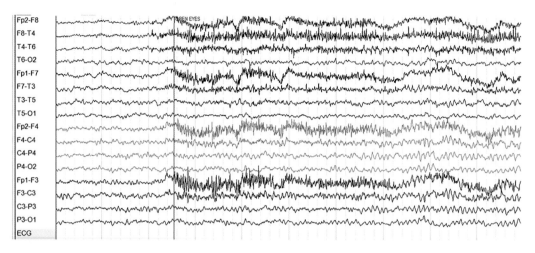

Figure 5.5   Paradoxical alpha during drowsiness. With eye opening (red vertical line), the posterior dominant alpha rhythm becomes more pronounced.

Mu rhythm

Similar to the alpha rhythm, mu is another reactive and normal rhythm in wakefulness found in 10–20% of the adult population on visual analysis of the EEG. The frequency is 7–12 Hz and slightly faster than the alpha rhythm of the individual. The morphology is characterized by a sharp negative phase and a rounded positive phase, giving rise to its typical "comb-like" and arciform shape. It is most prominent over the central region with the maxima involving C3 and C4 electrodes (Figure 5.6). Though bilateral in the majority, mu rhythm may demonstrate shifting from side to side. An exclusively unilateral mu rhythm is abnormal and raises the possibility of a lesion in the contralateral Rolandic region. The mu rhythm is typically attenuated by voluntary, passive, or reflex movements as well as tactile stimulation of the contralateral limbs. It has also been shown that the thought to move or imaginary movements of the contralateral limb attenuates the mu rhythm. Skull defects make mu more prominent and should be considered as a possibility when the mu rhythm is asymmetric.[6]

Beta rhythm

Beta rhythm typically consists of 14–30 Hz activity with amplitudes of <30 microvolts most prominent over the frontocentral regions during wakefulness.[7] It demonstrates reactivity very similar

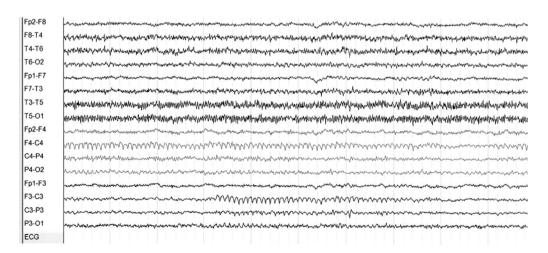

Figure 5.6   Mu rhythm. Note rhythmic arciform waveforms involving F4C4 and F3C3 electrodes.

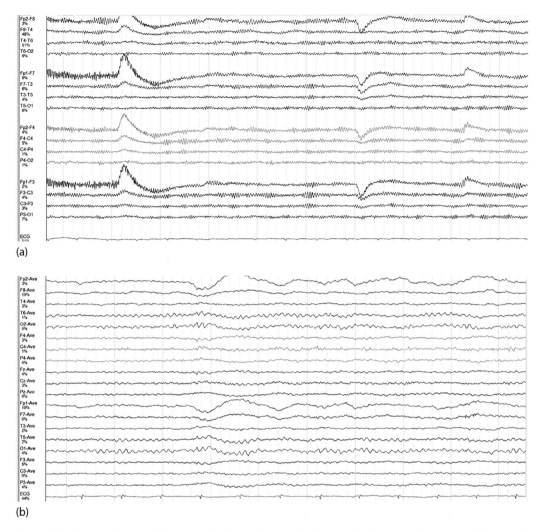

Figure 5.7   Beta rhythms. (a) Generalized beta activity recorded from a patient on benzodiazepines. (b) Persistent asymmetry in beta activity. Note in this sample of EEG in drowsiness (b), beta activity is seen over F4C4 but not on F3C3. This patient had a stroke in the left frontal region, which explains the asymmetric beta activity.

to mu whilst augmented by cognitive tasks such as mental arithmetic and light sleep.[6] Certain medications such as barbiturates, propofol, benzodiazepines, and neuroleptics tend to generate diffuse beta activity (Figure 5.7a).[6] Beta rhythm is typically symmetrical and consistently attenuated activity over a region or a hemisphere indicates an underlying structural abnormality or cortical dysfunction (Figure 5.7b).[6] Focally or regionally enhanced beta activity usually suggests a skull defect in the region.

Theta rhythm

It is normal to find a small amount of intermittent theta activity over the frontal and frontocentral regions during wakefulness. Theta activity becomes more prominent and prevalent with drowsiness and sleep. Intermittent, bilateral, and independent temporal theta activity can be a normal finding in individuals >50 years of age. Excessive theta activity and the presence of theta in the PDR are abnormal findings.

Lambda waves

Lambda waves are diphasic sharp transients with a dominant positive phase occurring over the occipital regions and elicited by saccadic eye movements due to the scanning of objects.

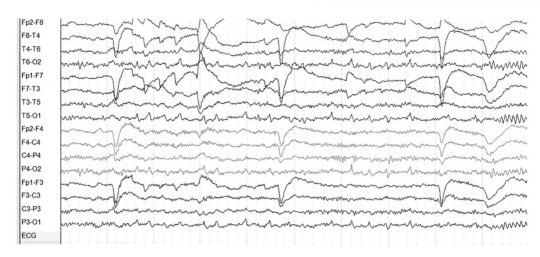

Figure 5.8   Lambda waves. Note eye movement artifacts anteriorly suggestive of scanning an object.

The amplitude is usually <50 microvolts.[7] The waves usually have a triangular shape and can be repetitive (Figure 5.8). Typically bilateral and synchronous, lambda waves are time-locked to saccadic eye movements. An alpha rhythm of >8.5 Hz is strongly correlated with lambda waves, and the presence of lambda waves is a significant predictor of normal EEG.[8]

NORMAL EEG IN SLEEP

A deep understanding of sleep stages and normal sleep-related EEG changes are very important for the electroencephalographer. Epileptiform discharges are more frequent in sleep. Meanwhile, normal sleep transients can be mislabeled as abnormal by a novice. Some paroxysmal changes during drowsiness can be particularly confusing. Detailed sleep stages are usually captured on prolonged ambulatory and video-EEG monitoring, though brief periods of sleep may be seen in routine and sleep-deprived EEGs.

It is useful to know some historical aspects of the visual scoring of sleep stages. The rules were developed in relation to polysomnography, rather than routine EEG. However, those rules are still applicable to our EEG practice as long as the technical differences in recording are kept in mind. First, polysomnography involves a lesser number of EEG electrodes – frontal to capture K-complexes and delta waves; central to capture theta activity, vertex waves, sleep spindles, and saw-tooth waves; and occipital to capture PDR. Second, there are electro-oculogram derivations to capture eye movements in polysomnography. In routine EEG, however, it is easy to incorporate extra electrodes to study eye movements, and those are particularly helpful to identify rapid eye movement (REM) sleep. Third, an EMG electrode over the chin is used in polysomnography to study muscle activity in scoring REM sleep. Finally, sleep scoring in polysomnography is epoch-based and each epoch is 30 seconds.

The first widely accepted sleep scoring rules were published by Rechtschaffen and Kales in 1968.[9] According to the R & K manual, sleep was divided into five stages: 1, 2, 3, 4, and REM. Table 5.1 summarizes the R & K scoring rules.[9] Stages 1 to 4 constitute non-rapid eye movement (NREM) sleep.

In 2007, the American Academy of Sleep Medicine (AASM) published updated scoring rules that are currently in use (Table 5.2).[10] Drowsiness is a term frequently encountered in EEG reports. It should be noted, that in sleep scoring, there is no stage called drowsiness. The transition from wakefulness to sleep is a continuum and drowsiness is within the sleep-wake boundary. For classification purposes, drowsiness is best considered to be aligned with sleep onset in the early stage N1 of sleep. Table 5.3 summarizes different sleep stages and corresponding findings.

Table 5.1 Rechtschaffen and Kales scoring rules (abbreviated)

Sleep stage	Scoring criteria
Waking	• >50% of the epoch contains 8–13 Hz alpha activity
1	• <50% of the epoch contains alpha activity • >50% of the epoch contains 2–7 Hz activity • Slow rolling horizontal eye movements
2	• Sleep spindles +/– K complexes • <20% of the epoch may contain high-voltage (>75 microvolts) low-frequency (<2 Hz) activity.
3	• 20–50% of the epoch contains high-voltage (>75 microvolts), low-frequency (<2 Hz) activity
4	• >50% of the epoch consists of high-voltage (>75 microvolts) low-frequency (<2 Hz) activity
REM	• EEG: Low voltage mixed (2–7 Hz) frequency • EYE: Episodic rapid eye movements • EMG: Absent or reduced chin EMG activity

Table 5.2 American Academy of Sleep Medicine scoring rules (abbreviated)

Sleep stage	Scoring criteria
W	• >50% of the epoch contains 8–13 Hz alpha activity/PDR

N1	• >50% of the epoch contains low-amplitude mixed-frequency (4–7 Hz) activity replacing alpha/PDR
	• Subjects who do not generate clear alpha rhythm:
	  a. 4–7 Hz activity
	  b. Slowing of stage W background frequencies by ≥1 Hz
	  c. Vertex sharp waves
	  d. Slow eye movements: Conjugate, regular, sinusoidal movements and initial deflection >0.5 seconds

N2	• 4–7 Hz low-amplitude mixed-frequency background • K complexes • Sleep spindles
N3	• >20% of the epoch contains 0.5–2 Hz slow activity of >75 microvolts peak-to-peak amplitude in the frontal derivation
R	• EEG: Low amplitude mixed frequency (4–7 Hz) • EOG: Rapid eye movements • EMG: Low chin-muscle tone

Table 5.3 Comparison of sleep stages and corresponding EEG markers

R & K	AASM	Key EEG features
Waking	Stage W	Alpha/PDR
Stage 1	Stage N1	Slow eye movements, positive occipital sharp transients of sleep (POSTS), vertex sharp waves
Stage 2	Stage N2	Sleep spindles, K complexes, (POSTS and vertex sharp waves may persist)
Stage 3	Stage N3	Synchronous high-amplitude delta (spindles may persist)
Stage 4	Stage N3	Synchronous high-amplitude delta (spindles fade)
Stage REM	Stage R	Rapid eye movements, sawtooth waves, low voltage mixed frequency, reduced muscle tone

Drowsiness and stage N1

As discussed, drowsiness is merged with stage N1 in a continuum and the separation is difficult and impractical. However, recognition of drowsiness and its spectrum of EEG patterns is an integral part of EEG reading. Hence, drowsiness is discussed with a particular emphasis next.

A reduction in muscle tone, as well as muscle and movement artifacts, is an early sign of drowsiness. Eye movements are particularly important to recognize drowsiness. The disappearance of eye blinks is the earliest recognizable sign of drowsiness. Eye blinks appear in two forms: high amplitude blinks when eyes are open and small amplitude blinks (mini blinks) with eyes closed. Both types disappear with the onset of drowsiness.[11] The hallmark of drowsiness is slow roving eye movements (Figure 5.9a). In the absence of electro-oculogram (EOG) electrodes, these movements can be recognized in frontal EEG derivations. Slow eye movements are sinusoidal, regular, and conjugate with the first shift from the baseline lasting >0.5 seconds.[10] Other motions such as small-fast-irregular eye movements and small-fast-rhythmic eye movements have been described in association with drowsiness.[11] However, those movements are difficult to capture with conventional EOG electrodes and need special motion transducers attached over the eyelid.

EEG changes in drowsiness can be broadly divided into two groups: transitional and post-transitional. The transition period refers to the brief gap before the alpha activity disappears. The post-transitional phase occurs after the alpha activity has disappeared.[11]

The key feature of the transitional phase is the change in alpha distribution and amplitude. During the transition, the alpha activity shifts from occipital to frontocentral or temporal regions, accompanied by an increase or decrease in amplitude (Figure 5.9b). Other notable changes are the

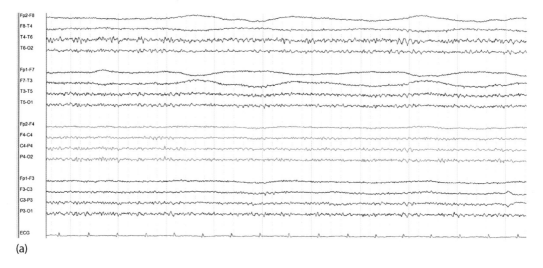

(a)

Figure 5.9a Slow horizontal eye movements of drowsiness.

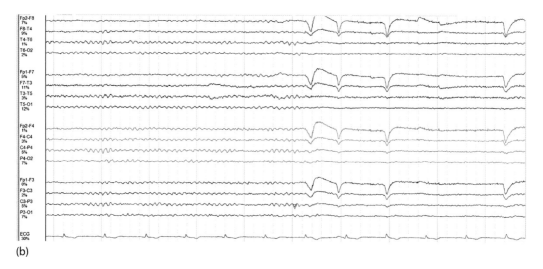

(b)

Figure 5.9b **Frontal migration of alpha during drowsiness.** Note how alpha rhythm disappears with eye blinks.

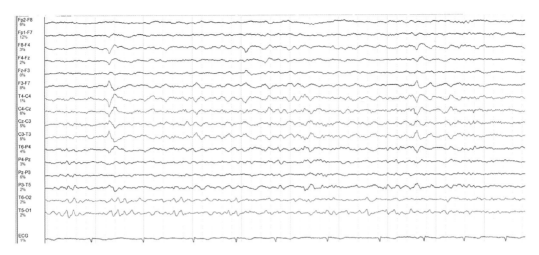

Figure 5.10 Vertex waves. Note parasagittal distribution is best visible on the transverse montage.

slowing of the alpha and the emergence of theta slowing in the frontocentral and temporal regions. Generalized attenuation of amplitudes and vertex sharp waves are recognized features during this stage. Vertex sharp waves (V waves) are high amplitude, diphasic transients with a prominent surface-negative wave followed by a small positive component lasing <0.5 seconds.[12] V waves are usually bilateral, symmetric, and synchronous with the amplitude maxima over the central (Cz) regions (Figure 5.10). Though they occur in isolation in adults, V waves can be asymmetric and appear in runs in children. V waves are generated spontaneously or in response to alerting stimuli.[12]

It is also important to recognize burst patterns that occur during the transitional phase to avoid mislabeling them as abnormal or epileptiform patterns. These bursts are characterized by sharply contoured, high amplitude, 2.5–7.5 Hz activity lasting 1–4 seconds with a frontocentral or generalized distribution.[11]

Typical post-transitional changes are positive occipital sharp transients of sleep (POSTS) and frontocentral slowing. As the name suggests, POSTS are triangular-shaped surface-positive transients with a steeper descending phase than the ascending phase over the occipital regions occurring in the form of single waves or a series.[12] POSTS usually last 80–200 msec with an amplitude of 20–75 microvolts (Figure 5.11). Though usually bilaterally symmetric and synchronous, asymmetries in

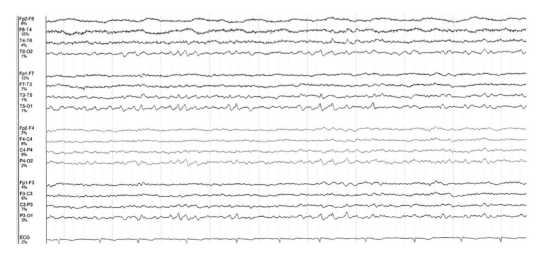

Figure 5.11 Positive occipital sharp transients of sleep.

POSTS are seen in normal subjects.[12] POSTS have a remarkably similar appearance to lambda waves. However, the differentiation is easy as lambda waves occur only in wakefulness in association with scanning eye movements.

Frontocentral beta activity and generalized 3–5 Hz slowing are seen in both the transitional and post-transitional phases. Several benign normal variants such as phantom spike waves, benign sporadic sleep spikes (BSSS), psychomotor variant, wicket waves, midline theta rhythm of Ciganek, 14 & 6 positive spikes, mitten pattern, and hypnogogic/hypnopompic hypersynchrony are also seen in drowsiness.[11] These normal variants will be discussed in Chapter 8.

Stage N2

EEG features of stage N2 are summarized in Table 5.2. The background shows generalized slowing consisting of 4–7 Hz low-amplitude mixed-frequency activity. K complexes and sleep spindles are hallmark graphoelements of N2 sleep. V waves and POSTS can continue into stage N2 from N1.

The K complex is defined by the AASM as a "well-delineated negative sharp wave immediately followed by a positive component standing out from the background EEG with total duration ≥0.5 seconds."[10] The maximum amplitude, ranging from 100 to 400 microvolts, is over the frontal regions.[13] Sometimes, the K complex is followed by a brief run of the alpha activity or a sleep spindle (Figure 5.12). There are two types of K complexes: spontaneous and those evoked by sensory stimuli. To score stage N2 sleep, at least one spontaneous K complex should be present during the first half of the epoch. If only K complexes associated with arousals occur, defined as arousal commencing within 1 second of the termination of the K complex, the epoch should be scored as stage N1.[10]

Sleep spindles are defined by the AASM as "a train of distinct waves with frequency 11–16 Hz (most commonly 12–14 Hz) with a duration ≥0.5 seconds, usually maximal in amplitude over the central regions."[10] There is no amplitude criterion, but is considered to be <50 microvolts.[12] As the name suggests, the spindle consists of a series of waveforms with gradually increasing and then decreasing amplitudes (Figure 5.13). Sleep spindles are usually bilaterally symmetric and synchronous. Persistently attenuated and/or slower spindles on one side suggest an underlying pathology in the hemisphere.[14] Based on the frequency and the distribution, two types of sleep spindles have been identified: slow (12–14 Hz, frontal) and fast (14–16 Hz, parietal).[15] From the cognitive neuroscience point of view, sleep spindles show a positive correlation with intellectual function and memory consolidation.[16]

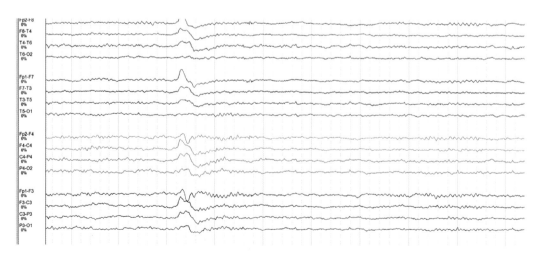

Figure 5.12 K complex.

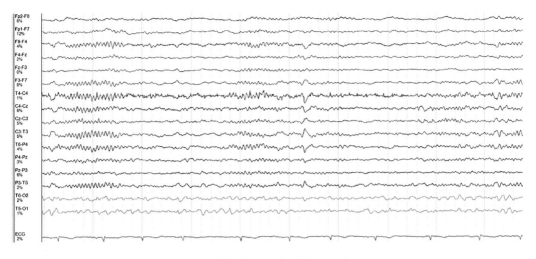

Figure 5.13 **Sleep spindles.** Visible in the first 2 seconds of the epoch.

Stage N3

The stage N3 or slow-wave sleep is characterized by 0.5–2 Hz high-amplitude delta activity of >75 microvolts (peak-to-peak amplitude) over the frontal region occupying >20% of the epoch (Figure 5.14).[10] Sleep spindles and K complexes may continue into stage N3 from N2. Growth hormone secretion peaks during this stage.[17] Many parasomnias typically occur during stage N3 and this period of sleep has the highest threshold for arousal.

Stage R (REM sleep)

The AASM rules require fulfillment of three features to score stage R: (1) Rapid eye movements, (2) attenuated chin muscle (EMG) tone, and (3) low-amplitude, mixed-frequency background. If those key phenomena are equivocal, phasic muscle twitches and sawtooth waves are considered supportive evidence.[10] Phasic muscle twitches are characterized by irregular EMG bursts lasting <0.25 seconds occurring on a background of low muscle tone. Sawtooth waves are triangular-shaped transients of 2–6 Hz frequency with amplitude maxima over Cz and Fz electrodes. Rapid eye movements are irregular but conjugate with a sharp peak and the first shift from the baseline lasts <0.5 seconds (Figure 5.15).[10] The muscle tone reaches the minimum during REM sleep.

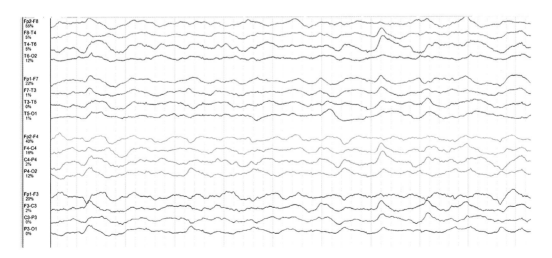

Figure 5.14 Slow-wave sleep.

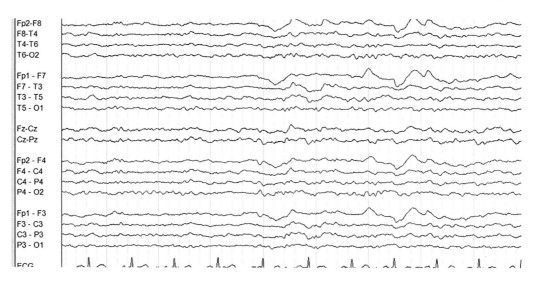

Figure 5.15   REM sleep. Note the artifact generated by rapid eye movements visible on anterior channels.

Sustained muscle activity is abnormal during REM sleep and the REM sleep behavior disorder is characterized by vivid dreams and excessive, often violent, movements related to the dream.

EEG arousals

The EEG arousal is defined as "an abrupt shift in EEG frequency which may include theta, alpha, and/or frequencies greater than 16 Hz but not spindles."[18] Furthermore, the shift should last ≥3 seconds with ≥10 seconds of sleep preceding the onset of the arousal. In NREM sleep, the arousals may or may not accompany an increase in the chin EMG amplitude. On the contrary, such an increase is a requirement to score arousal from REM sleep.

Major body movements

Body movements do occur during sleep, posing a challenge in scoring due to artifacts generated. If the movement occupies >50% of the epoch, it is scored as movement time according to the R & K scheme. However, this practice has been abandoned in AASM scoring rules. If the epoch with body movement artifact also shows alpha PDR, the epoch in question is scored as W (wakefulness). If not, it is scored the same as the staging of the next epoch.[10]

References

1. Petersen, I, Eeg-Olofsson, O. The development of the electroencephalogram in normal children from the age of 1 through 15 years. Non-paroxysmal activity. Neuropadiatrie 1971;2:247–304.

2. Duffy, FH, Albert, MS, McAnulty, G, Garvey, AJ. Age-related differences in brain electrical activity of healthy subjects. Ann Neurol 1984;16:430–438.

3. Storm Van Leeuwen, W, Bekkering, DH. Some results obtained with the EEG-spectrograph. Electroencephalogr Clin Neurophysiol 1958;10:563–570.

4. Adams, A. Studies on the flat electroencephalogram in man. Electroencephalogr Clin Neurophysiol 1959;11:35–41.

5. Westmoreland, BF, Klass, DW. Defective alpha reactivity with mental concentration. J Clin Neurophysiol 1998;15:424–428.

6. Kozelka, JW, Pedley, TA. Beta and mu rhythms. J Clin Neurophysiol 1990;7:191–207.

7. Kane, N, Acharya, J, Benickzy, S, et al. A revised glossary of terms most commonly used by clinical electroencephalographers and updated proposal for the report format of the EEG findings. Revision 2017. Clin Neurophysiol Pract 2017;2:170–185.

8. Tatum, WO, Ly, RC, Sluzewska-Niedzwiedz, M, Shih, JJ Lambda waves and occipital generators. Clin EEG and Neurosci 2013;44:307–312.

9. Rechtschaffen, A, Kales, A A Manual of Standardized Terminology Techniques and Scoring System for Sleep Stages of Human Subjects. Washington, DC: US Government Printing Office, 1968.

10. Silber, MH, Ancoli-Israel, S, Bonnet, MH, et al. The visual scoring of sleep in adults. J Clin Sleep Med 2007;3:121–131.

11. Santamaria, J, Chiappa, KH The EEG of drowsiness in normal adults. J Clin Neurophysiol 1987; 4:327–382.

12. Erwin, CW, Somerville, ER, Radtke, RA A review of electroencephalographic features of normal sleep. J Clin Neurophysiol 1984;1:253–274.

13. Bremer, G, Smith, JR, Karacan, I Automatic detection of the K-complex in sleep electroencephalograms. IEEE Trans Biomed Eng 1970;17:314–323.

14. Reeves, AL, Klass, DW Frequency asymmetry of sleep spindles associated with focal pathology. Electroencephalogr Clin Neurophysiol 1998;106:84–86.

15. Merica, H Fast and slow frequency spindles in sleep: Two generators? Clin Neurophysiol 2000; 111:1704–1706.

16. Fogel, SM, Smith, CT The function of the sleep spindle: A physiological index of intelligence and a mechanism for sleep-dependent memory consolidation. Neurosci Biobehav Rev 2011;35:1154–1165.

17. Holl, RW, Hartman, ML, Veldhuis, JD, Taylor, WM, Thorner, MO Thirty-second sampling of plasma growth hormone in man: Correlation with sleep stages. J Clin Endocrinol Metab 1991;72:854–861.

18. American Sleep Disorders Association. EEG arousals: Scoring rules and examples: A preliminary report from the Sleep Disorders Atlas Task Force of the American Sleep Disorders Association. Sleep 1992; 15:173–184.

CHAPTER 6

Activation techniques

Several activation procedures are employed during electroencephalogram (EEG) recording to increase the diagnostic yield. Hyperventilation (HV) and photic stimulation (PS) are routinely used. Sleep induction and sleep deprivation can also be considered activation techniques in selected patients.

HYPERVENTILATION

During a 3-minute period of hyperventilation, the partial pressure of carbon dioxide (pCO_2) level continues to drop reaching the nadir 30 seconds after ceasing HV, followed by a gradual return to the baseline in five minutes. In parallel, the partial pressure of oxygen (pO_2) increases during HV.[1] Systemic hypocapnia leads to cerebral vasoconstriction and reduced cerebral blood flow, causing a transient reduction in glucose and oxygen in the brain. These changes are thought to be the underlying mechanism of HV-related EEG slowing. HV also activates epileptiform EEG abnormalities, most probably through a separate and independent mechanism.[2] The American Clinical Neurophysiology Society recommends routine HV during EEG recordings for a minimum of 3 minutes followed by continued recording for >1 minute post-HV unless there is a contraindication, inability to perform, or poor compliance.[3] Usual contraindications for HV include recent stroke, significant respiratory or cardiovascular disease, recent intracranial hemorrhage, and sickle cell disease or trait.

Normal response

The normal HV response is characterized by a gradual buildup of generalized and synchronous slow-wave activity. It usually starts in the theta range and progresses to high-amplitude delta slowing (Figure 6.1). The extent of changes depends on several variables. First and foremost, the degree of hypocapnia, hence the degree of hyperventilation, is a crucial factor.[4] Age is another determinant with 70% of healthy children and <10% of healthy adults showing normal HV response.[5] The HV response tends to decline with age and the most marked response is seen from 8 to 12 years of age.[6] Hypoglycemia accentuates HV-induced slowing, whereas hyperglycemia has the opposite effect.[7] HV response is more prominent in the sitting position compared with supine posture.[8]

Abnormal response

After cessation of HV, slow waves disappear and the EEG usually returns to the baseline within 60 seconds. Prolonged HV response is seen in hypoglycemia and more commonly, in routine

DOI: 10.1201/9781003353713-8

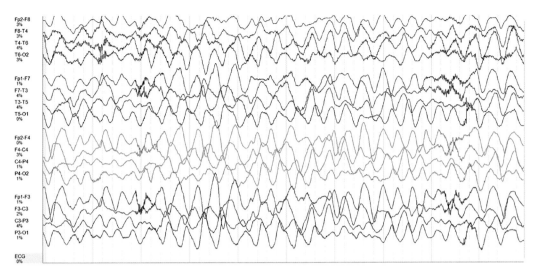

Figure 6.1 Normal hyperventilation response in a child. Note the symmetrical high-amplitude delta slowing.

recordings, when the subject continues to hyperventilate undetected by the technologist despite being requested to stop. In moyamoya disease, a "re-buildup" of slow-wave activity is seen up to 5 minutes after cessation of HV.[9]

The most useful clinical application of HV is to induce absence seizures, which will be discussed in more detail in Chapter 10. Hyperventilation can also trigger focal seizures and interictal epileptiform discharges (focal and generalized). Epileptiform discharges are activated more frequently (80%) in idiopathic generalized epilepsies compared with focal epilepsies (6–9%).[2] In drug-resistant focal epilepsy, 25% of patients demonstrated activation of focal seizures during 5 minutes of HV in the epilepsy monitoring unit setting.[2] Most seizures occurred during the fourth minute of HV, and at least 5 minutes of HV may be required to induce focal seizures.[2] Lateralized slowing is witnessed during HV among patients diagnosed with focal epilepsy syndromes.[10]

Non-epileptiform abnormalities such as accentuation of focal slowing, syncope, and psychogenic non-epileptic seizures are also triggered by HV.

INTERMITTENT PHOTIC STIMULATION

Intermittent photic stimulation (IPS) involves the delivery of trains of flashes with varying frequencies during eye closure, eyes closed, and eyes open states. Given the variability in the methodology used in different laboratories, an algorithm for IPS has been published with a view to standardizing the protocols.[11] The EEG may not show any change during the IPS. The IPS-triggered changes may or may not be clinically significant as listed next.

Photic driving

The photic driving response is characterized by rhythmic EEG activity over the posterior head regions triggered by IPS and time-locked to the photic stimulus (Figure 6.2). It is usually elicited with IPS frequencies of 5–30 Hz and most commonly around the alpha frequency of the subject. The photic driving frequency is usually identical to the IPS frequency, but can also occur in subharmonic (e.g., 50% of IPS frequency) or supraharmonic (two or three times the IPS) frequencies

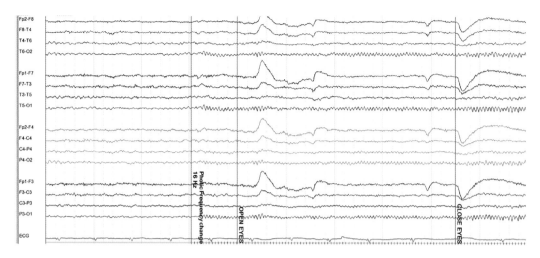

Figure 6.2   Normal photic driving response time-locked to the photic stimulus.

(Figures 6.3 and 6.4). Bilateral and symmetric photic driving is a normal finding. Consistently suppressed photic driving in a hemisphere, particularly in combination with focal slowing, may suggest an underlying structural abnormality.[12]

High-amplitude evoked spikes

Bi-occipital and symmetric high-amplitude (>100 microvolt) spikes are seen at low stimulation frequencies (<5 Hz) in patients with diffuse encephalopathies, including ceroid lipofuscinosis, neurodegenerative diseases, renal failure, and hepatic encephalopathy (Figure 6.5). These patients usually do not demonstrate photic driving at faster frequencies.[12]

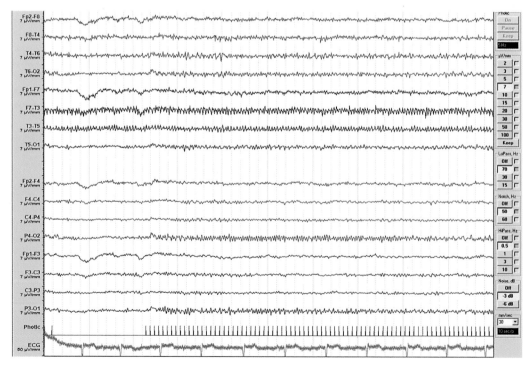

Figure 6.3   **Normal photic driving response supraharmonic to the photic stimulus.** The photic frequency is 10 Hz and the photic driving frequency is 20 Hz.

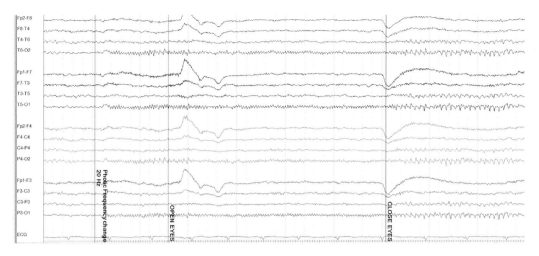

Figure 6.4   Normal photic driving response subharmonic to the photic stimulus. At 20 Hz photic stimulation, the first part of the EEG shows time-locked photic driving in synchrony, and the last 3 seconds following eye closure shows subharmonic (10 Hz) photic driving response.

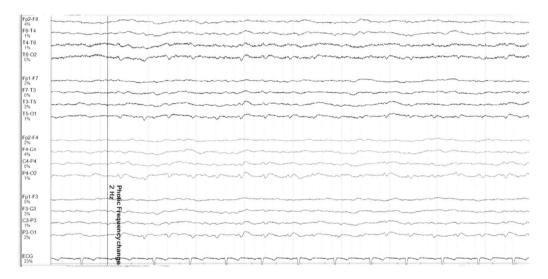

Figure 6.5   Occipital visual evoked response at 2 Hz photic stimulation time-locked to the stimulus in a patient with metabolic encephalopathy.

Electroretinogram

The electroretinogram (ERG) represents a retinal response to IPS and is captured by frontal (Fp1, Fp2) electrodes. This response can be distinctly seen in patients with electro-cerebral inactivity due to hypoxic brain injury (Figure 6.6).[13] The ERG complex is typically biphasic with a sharp "a" wave followed by a rounded "b" wave resembling a spike-wave complex. This phenomenon is most probably due to retinal cells being less susceptible to hypoxic injury than the cerebral cortex in the setting of hypoxic brain injury.[13] In hypoxic encephalopathy, it is important to avoid misinterpretation of ERG as cerebral reactivity, as it simply represents the local response from the surviving retinal cells. It can be seen in healthy individuals (Figure 6.7). Covering an eye during IPS will abolish the ipsilateral ERG.

Photomyogenic response

The photomyogenic response (PMR) is essentially an EMG artifact generated in the frontalis and orbicularis oculi muscles with IPS. PMR is usually triggered by IPS frequencies ranging

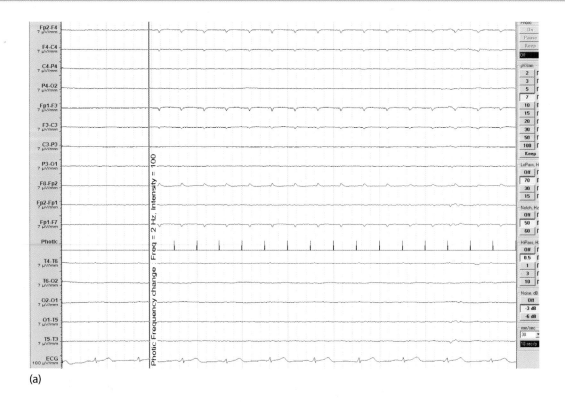

(a)

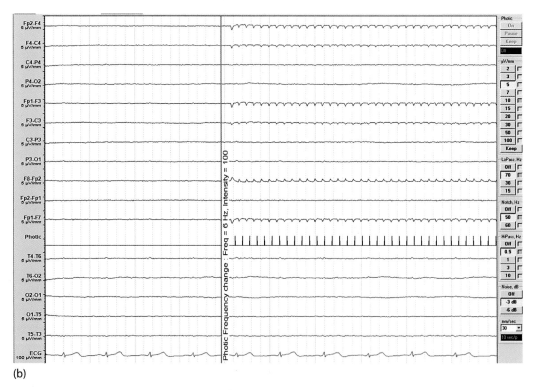

(b)

Figure 6.6a, b & c   Electroretinogram recorded from a patient with severe hypoxic encephalopathy. Note time-locked response maximum on Fp1 and Fp2 at multiple frequencies (a, b, & c) of photic stimulation. The generalized background suppression with amplitudes <10 microvolts indicates severe hypoxic brain injury. *(Continued)*

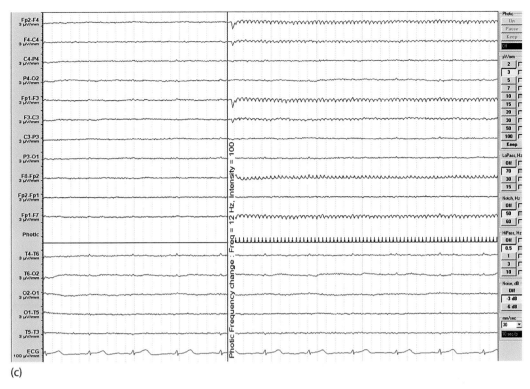

(c)

Figure 6.6   *(Continued)*

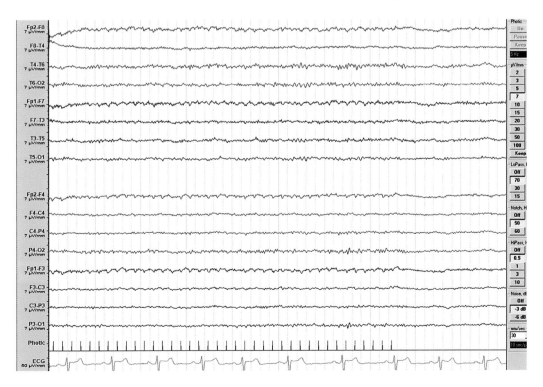

Figure 6.7   Electroretinogram recorded from an individual referred with a suspected seizure. Note the time-locked response maximum on Fp1 and Fp2.

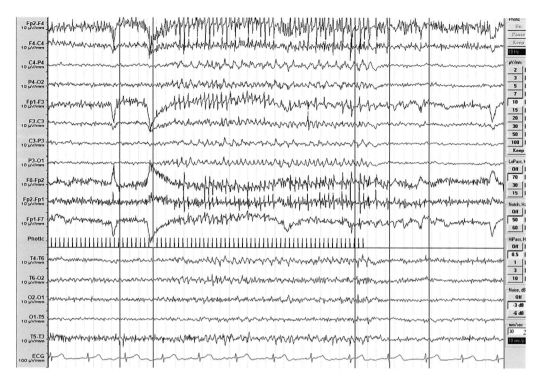

Figure 6.8   Photomyogenic response. Note the time-locked muscle artifact maximum at Fp1 and Fp2.

from 8 to 20 Hz (Figure 6.8).[14] The amplitude of the muscle artifact tends to gradually increase with the train of IPS. In some instances, the muscle activity may spread to other muscles in the head and neck region. However, the onset and offset are always time-locked with that of IPS. The photomyogenic response is often accompanied by visible eyelid flutter, vertical eyeball oscillations, and twitching of facial and neck muscles.[15] It should not be misdiagnosed as seizure activity. Though some old literature suggests that PMR is often seen during alcohol withdrawal, one study found it in only 4% of cases during acute alcohol withdrawal.[16] In summary, PMR is a non-specific finding with no clinical significance.

Photoelectric response

The photoelectric response is an electrode artifact generated by the local photochemical reaction of the electrode directly facing the photic stimulator, which acts as a photic cell when stimulated by the light. It appears as transient spikes over the electrode time-locked with the light stimulus and disappears when the electrode is covered to block the photic stimulation.

Photoparoxysmal response

The photoparoxysmal response (PPR) is the most important EEG abnormality characterized by polyspikes, polyspike-wave discharges, or spike-wave complexes triggered by IPS.[17] It is typically elicited by stimulus frequencies ranging from 15 to 20 Hz. PPR is usually seen in generalized epilepsies and rarely in focal epilepsies. It is also important to note that PPR may be detected in 0.3–4% of healthy adults without epilepsy.[18,19] The PPR is under the influence of several variables including age, sex, ethnicity, genetics, antiepileptic medication use, state of vigilance (sleep versus wakefulness), sleep deprivation, and the stimulation technique.

The two key elements in classifying PPR are the distribution and the temporal relationship to the stimulus. Several classifications of PPR are in use. Waltz et al. proposed four grades of PPR

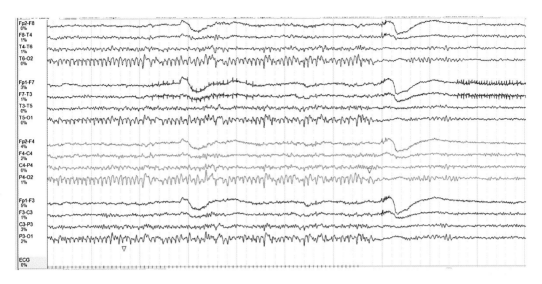

Figure 6.9   Type 1 photoparoxysmal response. Note the time-locked occipital response at 12 Hz. The photic stimulation frequency is 12 Hz.

ranging from occipital to generalized distribution.[20] Subsequently, three types of PPR have been described.[14]

1. Posterior stimulus-dependent response: These are high-amplitude visual evoked responses time-locked to the stimulus. In contrast to photic driving response, the waveforms have a sharp morphology. This response is observed in subjects with epilepsy as well as without (Figure 6.9).[21]

2. Posterior stimulus-independent response: Epileptiform patterns emerge in the posterior head regions with IPS but not at the flash frequency or harmonics of IPS (Figure 6.10). The activity may cease when the stimulus is terminated ("stimulus-limited") or persist beyond the point of flash termination ("self-sustained"). The response is defined as "self-sustained" when the EEG activity outlasts the stimulus by ≥100 ms.[22]

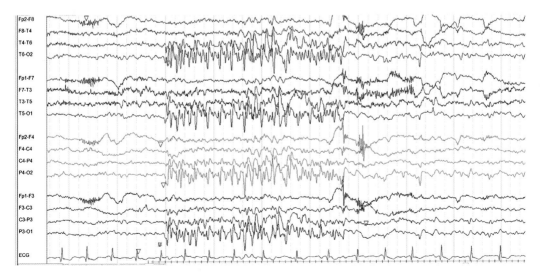

Figure 6.10   Type 2 photoparoxysmal response. Note the occipital response independent of the photic stimulation. The photic stimulation frequency is 8 Hz. A flicker is visible at the bottom of the EEG epoch.

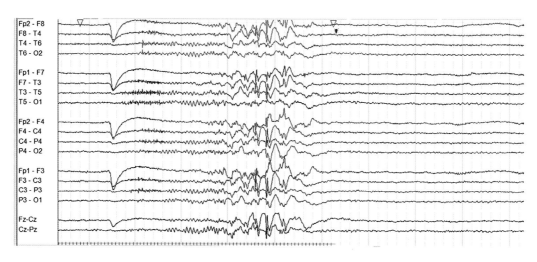

Figure 6.11   Type 3 photoparoxysmal response (stimulus-limited). Note the generalized photoparoxysmal response at 14 Hz of photic stimulation. The discharges do not extend beyond stimulation.

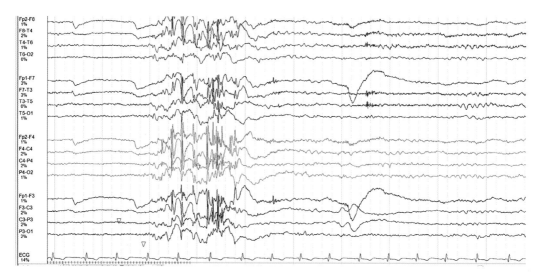

Figure 6.12   Type 3 photoparoxysmal response (self-sustained). Note the generalized photoparoxysmal response at 16 Hz of photic stimulation. The discharges continue beyond stimulation.

3. Generalized response: In generalized PPR, the distribution is generalized, but the maxima can be frontal or occipital. The temporal relationship to the IPS can be "stimulus-limited" or "self-sustained" (Figures 6.11 and 6.12). This is the typical response witnessed in idiopathic generalized epilepsies.

Activation of pre-existing epileptogenic networks

IPS may trigger clinical or electrographic seizures from pre-existing seizure networks, both focal and generalized, though it is not classified under the rubric of PPR (Figure 6.13a & b). The focus may be located within or outside the occipital cortex.

Psychogenic non-epileptic seizures

Occasionally, psychogenic non-epileptic seizures are triggered during IPS.[23] The EEG during the event demonstrates muscle and movement artifacts but no epileptiform ictal rhythm. The EEG reader must be aware of this possibility to avoid misdiagnosis.

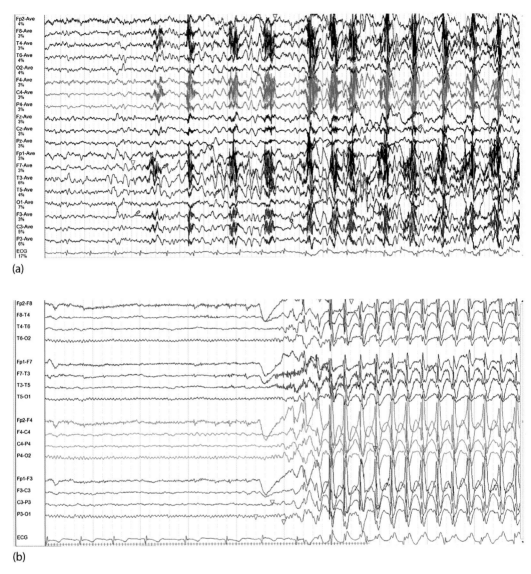

Figure 6.13 Activation of pre-existing epileptic networks during photic stimulation. (a) An electroclinical focal seizure is triggered by photic stimulation. Note the rhythmic activity build-up on F7 T3 spreading to Fp1 T5 and beyond as well as muscle artifacts due to oral automatisms. The time-base is compressed to 20 sec/page. Note the photic trigger displayed below the ECG channel. (b) An absence seizure triggered by photic stimulation. Note the photic trigger marked at the bottom of the figure (below the ECG channel).

PATTERN STIMULATION AND OTHER TRIGGERS

In reflex epilepsies, seizures are consistently triggered by various stimuli. Though not used routinely, such stimuli are useful to trigger epileptiform activity in selected patients during the EEG recording. Pattern sensitivity may occur in isolation or in combination with PPR. Striped patterns (square-wave gratings), with a spatial frequency between one and four cycles/degree are the most effective in eliciting an EEG response.[24] High brightness contrast, binocular vision, and larger patterns appear to increase the chances of triggering pattern sensitivity.[24]

Other reflex triggers include eating, video games, praxis, teeth brushing, being startled, music, board games, reading, decision making, and mental calculations.

Epileptiform discharges triggered by eye closure and fixation-off will be described in Chapter 10.

SLEEP AND SLEEP DEPRIVATION

Sleep can be considered an activation procedure as both focal and generalized epileptiform discharges increase in non-REM sleep. Seizures and epileptiform discharges are rare in REM sleep. The best technique to capture natural sleep is ambulatory EEG monitoring.[25] There is a significant increase in epileptiform discharges with sleep onset in idiopathic generalized epilepsies.[26] Similarly, two-thirds of epileptiform discharges occur in sleep in idiopathic generalized epilepsies.[25] Activation with sleep is particularly important and marked in certain epilepsy syndromes, such as benign Rolandic epilepsy, Landau-Kleffner syndrome, and continuous spike and wave during slow-wave sleep. In a study involving patients diagnosed with severe temporal lobe epilepsy, 30% had epileptiform discharges only during sleep.[27]

Sleep deprivation triggers epileptiform discharges as well as seizures. Many studies have reported an increased yield varying from 23% to 95% with total sleep deprivation.[28] However, making comparisons is very difficult due to wide variations in methodology and multiple confounding variables impacting the results. In idiopathic generalized epilepsies, sleep deprivation significantly increases the density of epileptiform discharges in both wakefulness and sleep, indicating sleep deprivation-related increase is independent of the sleep-related increase in epileptiform discharges.[29] Similar observations were reported from a mixed cohort of focal and generalized epilepsies.[30]

ANTISEIZURE DRUG WITHDRAWAL

Withdrawal of antiseizure drugs increases the chance of capturing seizures and interictal epileptiform discharges. Due to inherent risks, this activation procedure is recommended only for inpatients, particularly in the setting of epilepsy monitoring units.

References

1. Achenbach-Ng, J, Siao, TC, Mavroudakis, N, Chiappa, KH, Kiers, L. Effects of routine hyperventilation on PCO_2 and PO_2 in normal subjects: Implications for EEG interpretations. J Clin Neurophysiol 1994;11:220–225.

2. Guaranha, MSB, Garzon, E, Buchpiguel, CA, Tazima, S, Yacubian, EMT, Sakamoto, AC. Hyperventilation revisited: Physiological effects and efficacy on focal seizure activation in the era of video-EEG monitoring. Epilepsia 2005;46:69–75.

3. Sinha, SR, Sullivan, L, Sabau, D, San-Juan, D, Dombrowski, KE, Halford, JJ, et al. American Clinical Neurophysiology Society Guideline 1: Minimum technical requirements for performing clinical electroencephalography. J Clin Neurophysiol 2016;33:303–307.

4. Wirrell, EC, Camfield, PR, Gordon, KE, Camfield, CS, Dooley, JM, Hanna, BD. Will a critical level of hyperventilation-induced hypocapnia always induce an absence seizure? Epilepsia 1996;37:459–462.

5. Gibbs, FA, Gibbs, EL, Lennox, WG. Electroencephalographic response to overventilation and its relation to age. J Pediatr 1943;23:497–505.

6. Petersen, I, Eeg-Olofsson, O. The development of the electroencephalogram in normal children from the age of 1 through 15 years. Non-paroxysmal activity. Neuropadiatrie 1971;2:247–304.

7. Davis, H, Wallace, WM. Factors affecting changes produced in electroencephalogram by standardized hyperventilation. Arch NeurPsych 1942;47:606–625.

8. Billinger, TW, Frank, GS. Effects of posture on EEG slowing during hyperventilation. Am J EEG Technol 1969;9:22–27.

9. Kameyama, M, Shirane, R, Tsurumi, Y, Takahashi, A, Fujiwara, S, Suzuki, J, et al. Evaluation of cerebral blood flow and metabolism in childhood moyamoya disease: An investigation into "re-build-up" on EEG by positron CT. Childs Nerv Syst 1986;2:130–133.

10. Holmes, MD, Dewaraja, AS, Vanhatalo, S. Does hyperventilation elicit epileptic seizures? Epilepsia 2004;45:618–620.

11. Kasteleijn-Nolst Trenite, D, Rubboli, G, Hirsch, E, Martins da Silva, A, Seri, S, Wilkins, A, et al. Methodology of photic stimulation revisited: Updated European algorithm for visual stimulation in the EEG laboratory. Epilepsia 2012;53:16–24.

12. Coull, BM, Pedley, TA. Intermittent photic stimulation. Clinical usefulness of non-convulsive responses. Electroencephalogr Clin Neurophysiol 1978;44:353–363.

13. Wilkus, RJ, Chatrian, GE, Lettich, E. The electroretinogram during terminal anoxia in humans. Electroencephalogr Clin Neurophysiol 1971;31:537–546.

14. Kasteleijn-Nolst Trenite, DG, Guerrini, R, Binnie, CD, Genton, P. Visual sensitivity and epilepsy: A proposed terminology and classification for clinical and EEG phenomenology. Epilepsia 2001;42:692–701.

15. Kane, N, Acharya, J, Benickzy, S, Caboclo, L, Finnigan, S, Kaplan, PW, et al. A revised glossary of terms most commonly used by clinical electroencephalographers and updated proposal for the report format of the EEG findings. Revision 2017. Clin Neurophysiol Pract 2017;2:170–185.

16. Fisch, BJ, Hauser, WA, Brust, JC, Gupta, GS, Lubin, R, Tawfik, G, et al. The EEG response to diffuse and patterned photic stimulation during acute untreated alcohol withdrawal. Neurology 1989;39:434–436.

17. Chatrian, GE, Bergamini, L, Dondey, M, Klass, DW, Lennox-Buchthal, M, Petersen, I. A glossary of terms most commonly used by clinical electroencephalographers. Electroencephalogr Clin Neurophysiol 1974;37:538–548.

18. Gregory, RP, Oates, T, Merry, RT. Electroencephalogram epileptiform abnormalities in candidates for aircrew training. Electroencephalogr Clin Neurophysiol 1993;86:75–77.

19. Kooi, KA, Thomas, MH, Mortenson, FN. Photoconvulsive and photomyoclonic responses in adults. An appraisal of their clinical significance. Neurology 1960;10:1051–1058.

20. Waltz, S, Christen, HJ, Doose, H. The different patterns of the photoparoxysmal response–a genetic study. Electroencephalogr Clin Neurophysiol 1992;83:138–145.

21. Maheshwari, MC. The clinical significance of occipital spikes as a sole response to intermittent photic stimulation. Electroencephalogr Clin Neurophysiol 1975;39:93–95.

22. Puglia, JF, Brenner, RP, Soso, MJ. Relationship between prolonged and self-limited photoparoxysmal responses and seizure incidence: Study and review. J Clin Neurophysiol 1992;9:137–144.

23. Benbadis, SR, Johnson, K, Anthony, K, Caines, G, Hess, G, Jackson, C, et al. Induction of psychogenic nonepileptic seizures without placebo. Neurology 2000;55:1904–1905.

24. Wilkins, AJ, Darby, CE, Binnie, CD. Neurophysiological aspects of pattern-sensitive epilepsy. Brain 1979;102:1–25.

25. Seneviratne, U, Boston, RC, Cook, M, D'Souza, W. Temporal patterns of epileptiform discharges in genetic generalized epilepsies. Epilepsy Behav 2016;64:18–25.

26. Seneviratne, U, Lai, A, Cook, M, D'Souza, W, Boston, RC. "Sleep surge": The impact of sleep onset and offset on epileptiform discharges in idiopathic generalized epilepsies. Clin Neurophysiol 2020;131:1044–1050.

27. Niedermeyer, E, Rocca, U. The diagnostic significance of sleep electroencephalograms in temporal lobe epilepsy. Eur Neurol 1972;7:119–129.

28. Foldvary-Schaefer, N, Grigg-Damberger, M. Sleep and epilepsy: What we know, don't know, and need to know. J Clin Neurophysiol 2006;23:4–20.

29. Halasz, P, Filakovszky, J, Vargha, A, Bagdy, G. Effect of sleep deprivation on spike-wave discharges in idiopathic generalised epilepsy: A 4×24 h continuous long term EEG monitoring study. Epilepsy Res 2002;51:123–132.

30. Fountain, NB, Kim, JS, Lee, SI. sleep deprivation activates epileptiform discharges independent of the activating effects of sleep. J Clin Neurophysiol 1998;15:69–75.

CHAPTER 7

Artifacts
Generators, when to suspect, and how to resolve

Artifacts are unavoidable during electroencephalogram (EEG) recording and recognition of those is a critical step in EEG reading. Some artifacts may mimic brain activity, such as epileptiform discharges, whereas others mask underlying EEG activity, leading to misinterpretation.

Artifacts can be physiological (generated by the subject) or non-physiological (generated by the equipment and the environment). A good understanding of electrophysiological principles and technical aspects of EEG recording helps the reader detect these artifacts. The reader should ask a series of simple questions to separate true EEG signals from artifacts.

However, it must not be forgotten that artifacts can occasionally be very helpful. Eye-movement artifacts provide critical information about the state of vigilance. Ictal nystagmus can be easier to identify by way of eye-movement artifacts rather than the video. Increased muscle activity, particularly over the temporal regions, may indicate an anxious or tense patient. The appearance of a 60-Hz artifact on a channel during the EEG recording alerts the technologist that an input electrode has a high impedance that needs to be rectified. The emergence of biological artifacts in response to stimuli in a comatose patient may be early signs of improvement.

GENERATORS OF ARTIFACTS

Physiological

Eye movements

The eyeball is a dipole with an anterior positive charge (cornea) and a posterior negative charge (retina). Hence, eye movement generates a field captured by anterior electrodes depending on the direction of the movement as explained below.

a. When eyelids close, the eyeballs roll upward in keeping with the Bell's phenomenon. As a result, the frontal electrodes (Fp1, Fp2 > F3, F4) that are close to the eyeball capture a positive field. This field generates a downward deflection on the anterior channels of the longitudinal bipolar montage (Figure 7.1). An easy way to remember is that the deflection mimics the closing eyelids. Eye blink artifact is similar in shape and polarity but narrower in duration (Figure 7.1).

b. When eyes open, the opposite happens. The eyeballs roll downward and, as a result, the frontal electrodes (Fp1, Fp2 > F3, F4) capture a negative field because those electrodes are now closer to the negative end of the dipole (posterior part of the eyeball). The result is an upward deflection on the anterior channels of the longitudinal bipolar montage (Figure 7.1). An easy way to remember is that the deflection mimics eyelid opening.

c. Fast and subtle eyelid fluttering generates an undulating rhythmic theta- or alpha-like activity in the anterior leads (Figure 7.2a & b). This is known as the eye flutter artifact. The electrophysiological

DOI: 10.1201/9781003353713-9

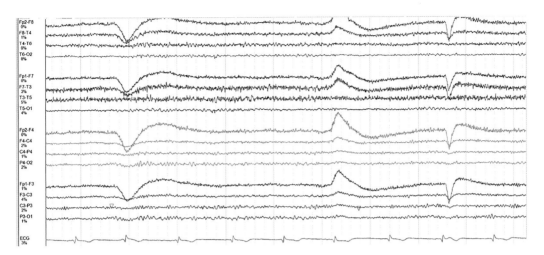

Figure 7.1   Eye-movement artifacts. The first downward deflection is consistent with eye closure, whereas the next upward deflection is caused by eye opening. The last downward deflection is due to an eye blink.

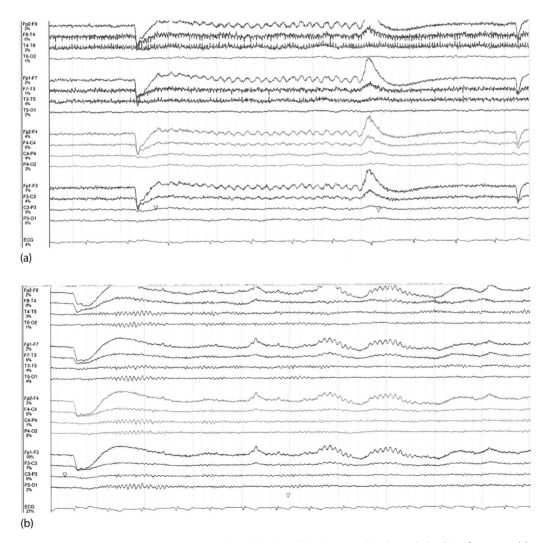

(a)

(b)

Figure 7.2   Eyelid flutter causing a rhythmic artifact involving the anterior channels in theta frequency (a). A similar artifact generates a faster artifact in the alpha range (b).

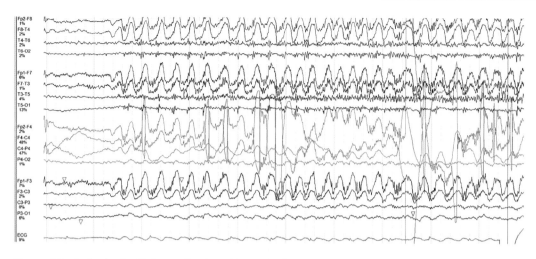

Figure 7.3   A rhythmic, high-amplitude, 3 Hz eyelid flutter artifact involving anterior EEG channels recorded during a psychogenic non-epileptic seizure. There are additional rhythmic movement artifacts in posterior head regions due to rhythmic head shaking.

explanation is similar to the artifact created by eye closure in (a) with repeated and fast rhythmic eyelid closures. Rhythmic eyelid flutter and repetitive blinking, particularly when admixed with muscle artifacts, can mimic epileptiform activity (Figure 7.3).

d. Lateral eye movements generate a different picture. If the subject is looking to the right, the positive end of the eyeball moves to the right. As a result, the right lateral and frontal electrodes (F8 > Fp2) capture the positive end of the dipole while the left lateral and frontal electrodes (F7 > Fp1) become negative. On a longitudinal bipolar montage, this particular field creates a positive phase reversal in the right anterior channels and a negative phase reversal in the left anterior channels. The exact opposite will be seen if the subject is looking to the left. Remember, the anterior channels "open up" when the person is looking in that direction (Figure 7.4).

e. With fast horizontal eye movements, as occurs in REM sleep and nystagmus, F7 or F8 electrodes may capture the muscle "twitch" of the lateral rectus muscle. This muscle artifact looks like a spike (rectus lateralis spike) (Figure 7.5).

Myogenic artifacts

The myogenic artifact appears in three forms:

1. Single muscle twitch: This is the equivalent of a single motor unit potential. The morphology may resemble an epileptiform spike. However, a careful evaluation will reveal several distinctive features. Muscle twitches appear over a specific muscle (e.g., frontalis, temporalis, lateral rectus) with a narrow field. They are usually diphasic or polyphasic without an aftercoming slow wave. The positive phase is more prominent than in epileptiform spikes (Figure 7.6). Repetitive muscle twitches can be mistaken for an ictal rhythm (Figure 7.6). However, the lack of evolution and individual characteristics of the muscle twitch units described above should help the reader make the distinction.

2. Burst pattern: The myogenic artifact appears in the form of repetitive bursts. Good examples are the chewing artifact and muscle artifact during the clonic phase of a seizure (Figure 7.7). Once again, the characteristics of the individual unit are very helpful to differentiate the artifact from epileptiform discharges. The muscle bursts are polyphasic with a high amplitude involving a specific region where the muscle is located and have a narrow field. In contrast to epileptiform discharges, there is no slow wave component. The positive phase is more prominent than in epileptiform spikes. When the burst pattern is admixed with rhythmic movement artifacts, as often happens, it may mimic an ictal rhythm. However, in contrast to a true ictal rhythm, the repetitive burst artifact does not evolve but often fluctuates.

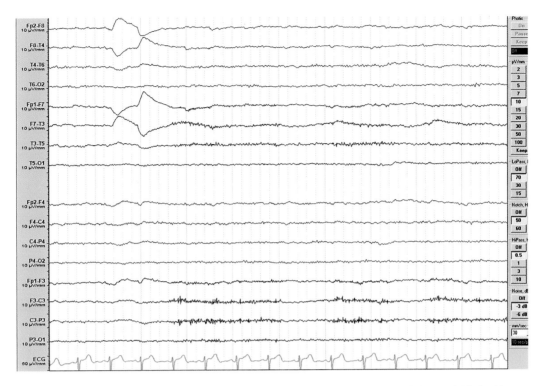

Figure 7.4   An eye-movement artifact generated by first looking to the right and then quickly looking to the left. Note the opposite polarities of the artifacts.

3. Tonic pattern: This is the equivalent of the full recruitment pattern in electromyography (EMG). With tonic muscle activation, a dense high-frequency artifact is visible over the involved muscles such as temporalis and frontalis (Figures 7.8 and 7.9a). When the timebase is expanded, it becomes clear that the artifact consists of closely packed spiky and polyphasic muscle potentials (Figure 7.9b). The subject is awake and usually tense. Lowering the high-frequency filer will reduce the artifact, but the remaining muscle activity resembles beta activity and can be misidentified as brain activity (Figure 7.10).[1]

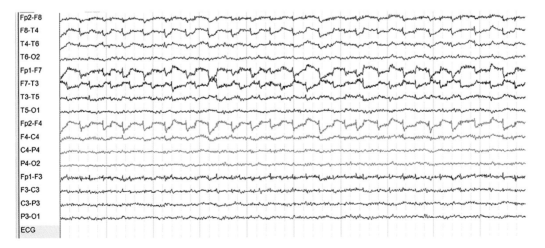

Figure 7.5   Eye-movement artifacts and rectus lateralis spikes generated by left-beating nystagmus. Note the rhythmic and fast horizontal eye movements accompanied by the artifact of lateral rectus muscles evident on anterior EEG channels.

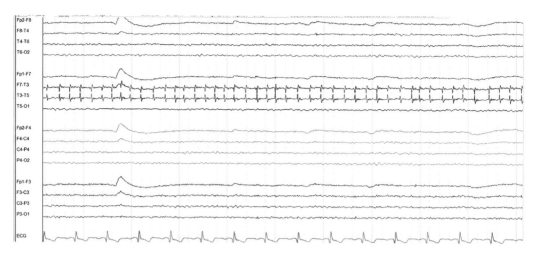

Figure 7.6   Artifact due to a single muscle twitch of the left temporalis muscle captured by the T3 electrode.

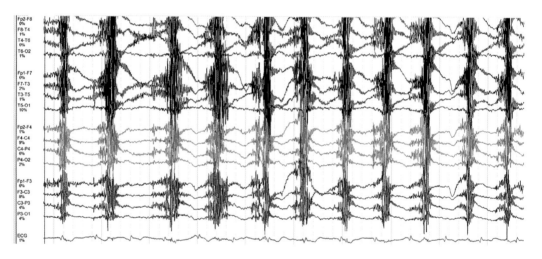

Figure 7.7   The burst pattern of muscle artifact generated by chewing.

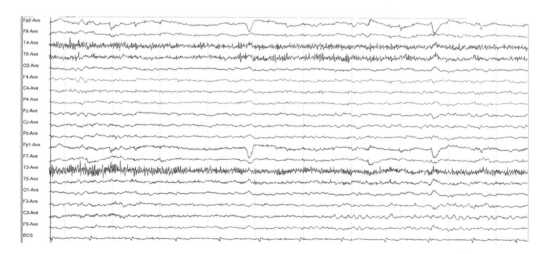

Figure 7.8   The tonic pattern of a muscle artifact generated by temporalis muscles and captured on T3, T4, and T6 electrodes.

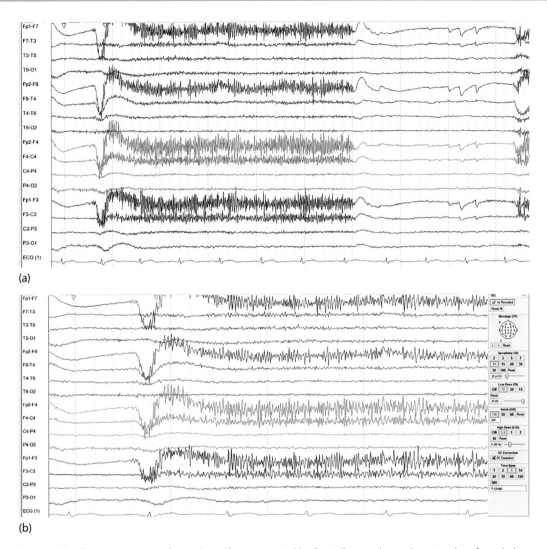

(a)

(b)

Figure 7.9 The tonic pattern of muscle artifact generated by frontalis muscles and captured on frontal electrodes (a). The expansion of the timebase to 5 seconds per page reveals the polyphasic morphology of the muscle artifact (b).

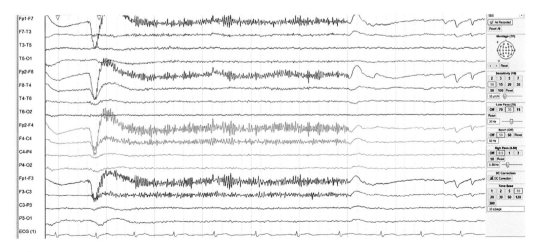

Figure 7.10 Lowering the high-frequency filter to 30 Hz gives the false impression of beta activity over those channels with muscle artifact in Figure 7.9.

The myogenic artifact is unavoidable in EEG recordings. In generalized tonic-clonic seizures, the myogenic artifact masks the underlying ictal rhythm. However, there are specific EMG signal patterns associated with tonic-clonic seizures, and those signal patterns acquired through surface EMG can be useful in seizure detection.[2] Furthermore, the surface EMG signal pattern can reliably differentiate convulsive epileptic seizures from psychogenic non-epileptic seizures.[3]

Glossokinetic artifacts

The tip of the tongue is negatively charged while the base is positive, thus acting as a bioelectric dipole. Tongue movements generate slow waves as a result of direct current potentials produced. The maxima and distribution of the field depends on the direction of movements; up-down, side-to-side, anterior-posterior, or a mix. The up-down movement (e.g., saying "lalalala") generates rhythmic delta slowing with bifrontal maxima (Figure 7.11). Side-to-side tongue movements generate rhythmic delta of temporal maxima (Figure 7.12). Glossokinetic artifacts generated during eating and talking are more complex but can be deduced by visualizing the dipole arrangement. When admixed with spike-like muscle artifacts, the glossokinetic artifact can be misidentified as epileptiform polyspike-wave activity.

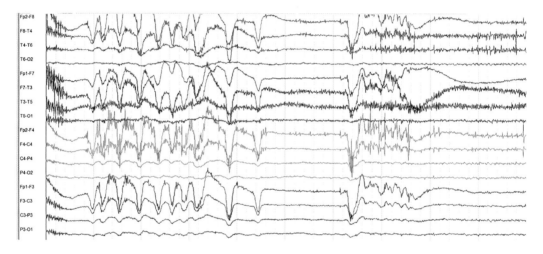

Figure 7.11   A glossokinetic artifact generated by up-down movements of the tongue.

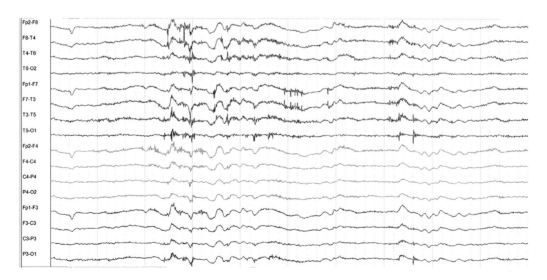

Figure 7.12   A glossokinetic artifact generated by lateral movements of the tongue.

Movement-related artifacts

Artifacts caused by movement arise from electrodes and their connecting lead wires. These artifacts are often admixed with muscle artifacts. Depending on the type of movement, the artifact may be rhythmic or arrhythmic. Rhythmic artifacts can be mistaken for an epileptiform ictal rhythm, but the lack of evolution usually helps to differentiate (Figure 7.13). Movement-related artifacts are particularly challenging in psychogenic non-epileptic seizures where different artifact patterns have been described.[4] The best approach to identify these artifacts is to carefully correlate them with the synchronous video recording.

Cardiac artifacts

1. *The ECG artifact:* This is generated by the QRS complex and depends on the vector direction. This is often seen in overweight or obese individuals with short necks. Temporal channels and referential montages, particularly ear reference, tend to accentuate the artifact while it is less prominent on bipolar montages. The ECG artifact may appear as periodic discharges on the EEG, but a vertical cursor confirming the one-to-one correlation with the QRS complex will solve the problem quite easily (Figure 7.14). The ECG artifact typically involves multiple channels equally and if it is more prominent in a single channel, the possibility of high electrode impedance should be raised.

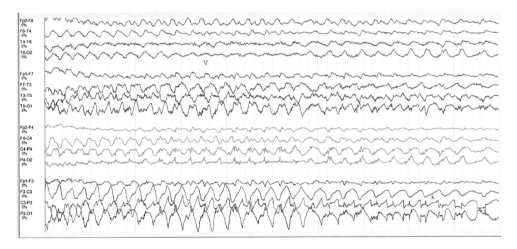

Figure 7.13 A rhythmic movement artifact caused by a psychogenic non-epileptic seizure. Note the multiple phase reversals, varying amplitudes, and the lack of evolution of rhythmic activity.

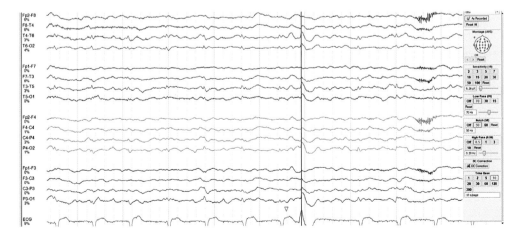

Figure 7.14 Widespread ECG artifact. Note that a ventricular ectopic (marked by a vertical cursor) generates an artifact of different morphology and amplitude on the EEG.

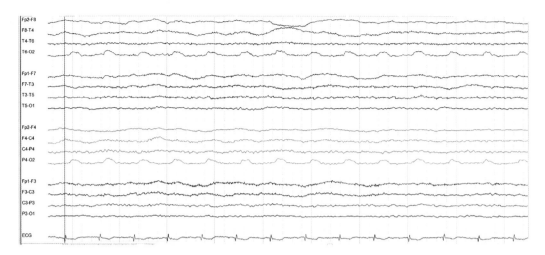

Figure 7.15   A pulse artifact captured by the right occipital electrode. Note slow-wave morphology, rhythmicity, and time-locked appearance after each QRS complex of the ECG.

2. *The pulse artifact:* When the electrode is placed over a small artery, the pulsation appears as rhythmic slow waves time-locked with the QRS complex occurring about 200 milliseconds after the QRS complex (Figure 7.15). Repositioning the head or slightly changing the electrode position during the recording can eliminate the artifact.

3. *The ballistocardiographic artifact:* Hyperdynamic circulation may cause slight head movements with vigorous cardiac contractions. It results in oscillation of the EEG leads, usually occipital, generating a rhythmic slow-wave artifact correlated with the ECG. It can be minimized by bundling the leads together.

Sweat artifacts

Sweat artifacts appear as high-amplitude and very low-frequency (<0.5 Hz) undulating waveforms involving multiple electrodes (Figure 7.16). Areas of the scalp with sweat glands are negatively charged compared with the rest, resulting in a voltage difference and generating electrical potentials.[5] Additionally, the chemical constituents in sweat change the skin resistance, and the electrolyte concentrations between the skin and the electrode with a battery-effect contribute to the slow-wave artifact.[5]

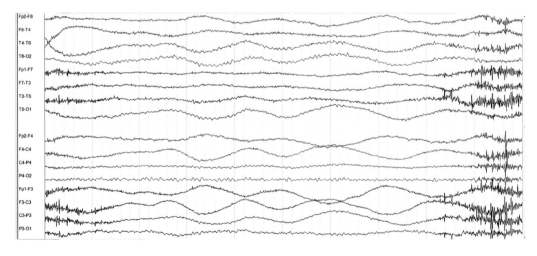

Figure 7.16   Sweat artifact.

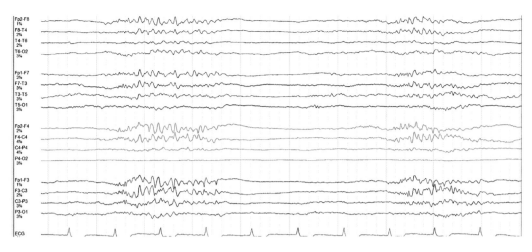

Figure 7.17   Bridging artifact. This EEG shows a burst suppression pattern. Note the P4-O2 channel is "flat" during bursts due to a salt bridge connecting the two electrodes.

Another impact of sweating is the creation of a "salt bridge." Sodium chloride in the sweat functions as a conductor between two electrodes "bridging" them so that the two electrodes of the particular channel become isopotential, manifesting as a (nearly) flat line on the EEG (Figure 7.17).

Sweat artifacts and bridging artifacts can be reduced by cooling the head with a fan or air conditioning and wiping the area with alcohol.

Non-physiological
Electrodes and connections
The electrode "pop" is the most frequent electrode artifact. Drying electrolytes or mechanical instability in the electrode-skin interphase results in an electrically unstable electrode that generates an electrode "pop."[5] Morphologically, it may sometimes resemble an epileptiform spike or sharp wave with a steep upstroke followed by a less-steep descent to the baseline (Figure 7.18a & b). The morphology may also resemble a slow wave and on a bipolar montage, the "pop" appears phase reversing (Figure 7.18c). Applying a referential montage will make it clear that it arises from a single electrode with no voltage field (Figure 7.18d). Poor electrode contact may generate a rhythmic artifact (Figure 7.18e).

Each electrode is connected to amplifiers via the jackbox. If the electrode pin is plugged into the wrong receptacle of the jackbox, bizarre artifacts will appear as illustrated in Figure 7.19. Here, the ECG electrode is mistakenly plugged into the receptacle of T6 and vice versa, resulting in the ECG appearing on T6 (Figure 7.19a). When this swap is corrected, normal ECG and EEG activities can be seen over T6 and ECG channels (Figure 7.19b).

Electrodes with high impedance give rise to several artifacts including the 60 Hz artifact, which will be described later. Another important "artifact" due to high impedance is ground lead recording. As explained in Chapter 2, there are three electrodes connected to a channel; input 1, input 2, and the ground electrode. If input 1 or 2 have very high impedances, the ground electrode (usually placed over mid-forehead) becomes an active (input) electrode, giving rise to unusual waveforms. For example, in the T5-O1 channel, if the T5 electrode has a high impedance, the ground electrode takes its place and becomes an active input. Therefore, in effect, the channel reflects the G-O1 connection. As the ground electrode is over the forehead, it will capture the eye blink electrical field and the eye blink artifact appears posteriorly over the T5-O1 channel!

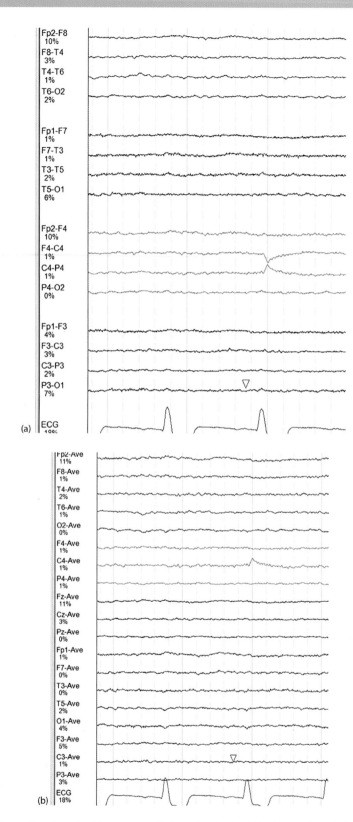

Figure 7.18 Electrode artifacts. (a) Sharp morphology, longitudinal bipolar montage. (b) Sharp morphology, common average reference montage. (c) Slow-wave morphology, longitudinal bipolar montage. (d) Slow-wave morphology, common average reference montage. (e) Rhythmic artifact generated by the F7 electrode due to poor contact. *(Continued)*

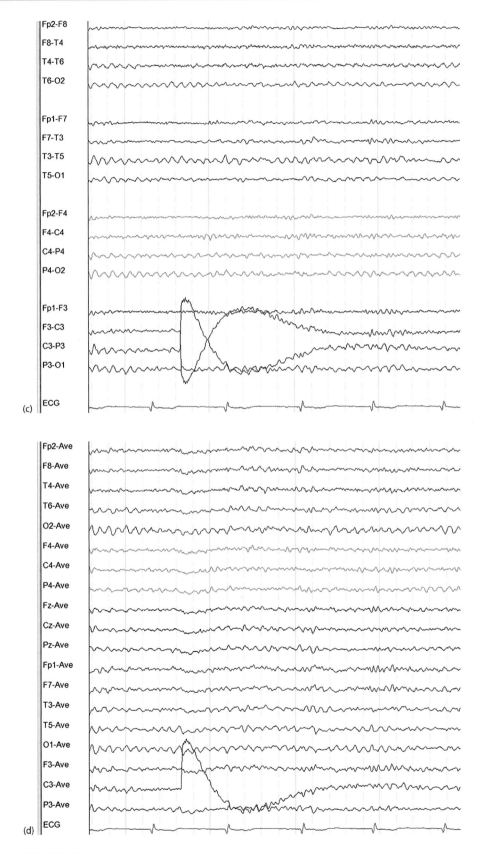

Figure 7.18 *(Continued)*

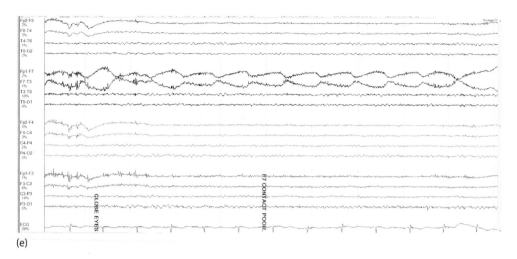

(e)

Figure 7.18   *(Continued)*

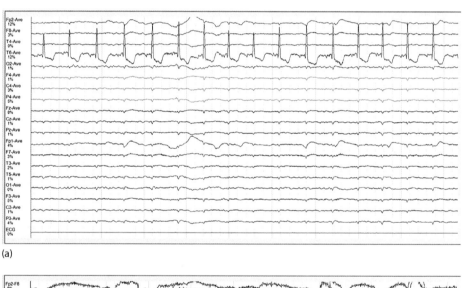

(a)

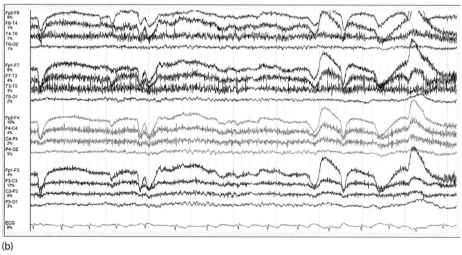

(b)

Figure 7.19   Artifact generated by electrode swap at the jackbox. (a) High-amplitude ECG artifact is visible at T6 on the common average reference montage with reduced amplitude by changing the sensitivity. (b) Normal EEG and ECG appearance after rectifying the swap.

Mains power supply (50 Hz/60 Hz) artifacts

The alternating electrical interference from the mains power supply with a frequency of 60 Hz (North and South America, Canada) or 50 Hz (Europe, Australia, Asia) generates this well-known artifact. Both electrostatic and electromagnetic interferences can cause the 60 Hz artifact. However, this is usually minimal with proper grounding and has a trivial impact on the EEG due to common-mode rejection. If one electrode has a high impedance, the 60 Hz artifact appears in the channel due to an imbalance between the two electrodes (Figure 7.20).

A widespread 60 Hz artifact usually suggests high impedances of the ground or reference electrodes or faulty grounding of the EEG machine (Figure 7.21). If 60 Hz artifact appears during the recording, the technologist should check the impedance of the particular electrode and rectify it. If the artifact appears in all channels, the technologist should check the impedances of the ground and reference electrodes immediately.

Removing the 60 Hz artifact is easy at the reviewing stage by applying the notch filter. However, during the recording, the notch filter should not be applied as the appearance of the 60 Hz artifact alerts the technologist regarding electrodes with high impedance and electrical safety.[1]

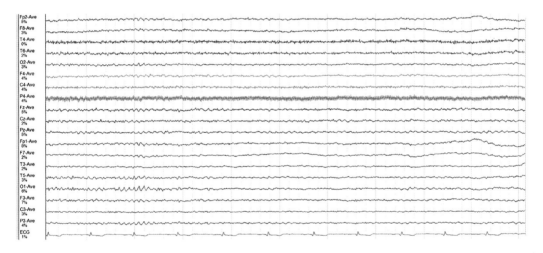

Figure 7.20   A 50-Hz artifact involving a single EEG channel. A common average reference montage. Note the 50-Hz artifact involving the P4 electrode due to its high impedance.

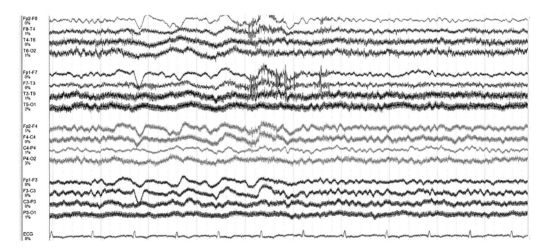

Figure 7.21   Widespread 50-Hz artifact due to high impedance of the ground electrode.

Instrumental artifacts

Malfunctions of different parts of the EEG machine can give rise to artifacts. Artifacts caused by electrodes and connectors have already been discussed. Malfunctioning amplifiers can generate a high-amplitude noise that may distort EEG waveforms. Aliasing artifacts during analog-to-digital conversion and the signal display have been described in a previous chapter. The "Blocking artifact" occurs due to amplifier saturation, whereas the "multiplexing artifact" is caused by sampling only a proportion of channels connected to the amplifier.[6]

Environmental artifacts

EEG recordings are particularly susceptible to artifacts in certain environments such as intensive care units where multiple signal generators (such as ventilators, cardiac monitors, and infusion pumps) run simultaneously.

Electrostatic artifacts are generated from mains electrical cables and similar sources moving close to the patient undergoing EEG. When there are two conductors close to each other, alternating potential in one conductor induces a potential of opposite polarity in the other. The human body functions as a conductor. Movement of cables, wires, and even personnel close to the patient may generate electrostatic artifacts resembling spikes and slow waves.[5,6] Intravenous drips can induce an electrostatic artifact in the form of a transient with the movement of each drip.[5]

Other potential environmental sources of artifacts include electromagnetic induction, mobile phones, high-frequency equipment such as diathermy, sudden voltage fluctuations of the mains supply, faulty switches, and hospital paging systems.

Implanted stimulators

Implanted medical devices such as vagus nerve stimulators, deep brain stimulators, and spinal stimulators generate artifacts during stimulation. These artifacts tend to be widespread and of high amplitude with some resemblance to epileptiform discharges. Precise interdischarge interval and unvarying morphology suggest the signals are generated by a machine rather than the brain (Figure 7.22a & b).[6]

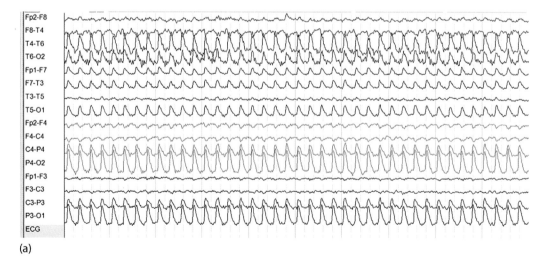

(a)

Figure 7.22 Artifact generated by deep brain stimulation in a patient with Parkinson's disease. (a) Note the widespread regular artifact with precise rhythmicity generated by the deep brain stimulator. (b) Once the device is turned off (mid-epoch), the EEG returns to its normal baseline instantly. *(Continued)*

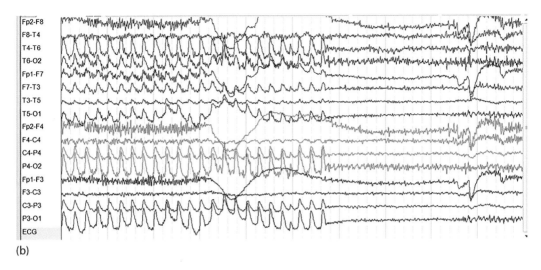

(b)

Figure 7.22 *(Continued)*

WHEN TO SUSPECT ARTIFACTS?

1. Waveforms are confined to a single electrode or a channel. EEG signals recorded from a true source should follow electrophysiological principles such as a voltage field and an electrical dipole. If the recorded signal does not conform to these rules, one must think about the possibility of an artifact. For example, a transient confined to a single electrode without a field should raise the suspicion of an artifact.[6] However, it must be remembered that the eye and the tongue are electrical dipoles, though the signals are classified as artifacts.

2. Waveforms are seen on multiple electrodes but do not follow a sensible electrophysiological field. The EEG reader must study the anatomical location of the electrodes. As discussed in a previous chapter, the amplitude is maximum at a certain point and gets smaller when moving away from the epicenter depending on the dipole orientation. If the field does not follow those electrophysiological rules, it is likely to be an artifact. Similarly, non-contiguous activity in a region when some electrodes skip the activity (e.g., waveform on Cz and T3, but not C3), an artifact should be suspected.

3. The appearance of complex waveforms. The reader must be familiar with the repertoire of waveforms usually encountered in practice. Most waveforms we see are mono-, di-, or triphasic. Muscle artifacts are often polyphasic. Unusual complex morphologies should raise the suspicion of an artifact.

4. Alternating multiple phase reversals involving adjacent electrodes. As discussed in a previous chapter, double phase reversals can be seen in the setting of an oblique dipole. However, alternating phase reversals in adjacent electrodes would be rather unusual and should raise the suspicion of an artifact.

5. Very high or very low frequencies. The brainwaves we are interested in usually appear within 1 Hz to 70 Hz. Muscle artifacts are of much higher frequencies. Very low frequencies of <0.1 Hz (infraslow activity) can be useful in the localization of epileptiform activity. However, more often, very slow frequencies represent artifacts such as sweat or movement artifacts.

6. Persistence of a specific frequency in a particular region. The best example is the 60 Hz artifact. This can be seen involving an electrode with a high impedance persistently.

7. Precise rhythmicity and periodicity. Rhythmic and periodic patterns are well recognized with brainwaves, but precise periodicity and rhythmicity should raise suspicion for artifacts generated by a machine.

8. The environment. EEGs recorded in the intensive care setting are particularly susceptible to artifacts. "Flat" EEGs, particularly in coma, tend to pick up artifacts from the environment. With numerous machines and equipment functioning simultaneously, EEG artifacts from those generators are not uncommon.

9. Pattern recognition. Some artifacts demonstrate characteristic morphologies and distribution. Eye blink artifacts have a specific morphology involving the frontal electrodes, whereas horizontal eye movements demonstrate a different morphology in the anterior leads. Chewing generates a very characteristic rhythmic artifact due to the combinations of masticatory muscle activity and tongue movements. The myogenic artifact is usually seen in electrodes over the temporalis and frontalis muscles. ECG artifacts have a sharp morphology time-locked to the QRS complex seen in the ECG channel. The pulse artifacts always follow the QRS complex of the ECG and are seen over the temporal or occipital artery.

HOW TO RESOLVE ARTIFACTS

Resolving artifacts occurs at two levels: the technologist and the reader. The technologist should identify artifacts during the recording and take measures to resolve or minimize the impact. When the reader suspects artifacts, parameters such as montages and sensitivities should be manipulated rationally to confirm and then remove artifacts.

EEG technologist

1. Check the impedance and re-gel the electrode. The appearance of the 60 Hz artifact on an electrode should alert the technologist to check the impedance and rectify the problem. Similarly, the appearance of electrode pops and similar artifacts should be dealt with by fixing the electrode.

2. Get the subject to relax. Muscle and movement artifacts indicate a tense and fidgety subject. The EEG technologist should talk to the subject, explain, and try to get the person to relax. Deep breathing is often an efficient way of relaxation. Recurrent eye blinks and eyelid flutter can be a problem in anxious and tense subjects. If relaxation does not work, eye patches may have to be applied to cover the eyes and reduce blinking.

3. Check electrodes and connections. The appearance of unusual and atypical waveforms should prompt the technologist to check the electrodes (particularly ground and reference) and connections. If the photoelectric response artifact is suspected, covering the particular electrode during photic stimulation eliminates the artifact and can be used as a test to confirm the origin of the artifact. Conversely, the electroretinogram is abolished by covering the eye. If an artifact confined to a single electrode is encountered, the first step is to reapply the electrode. If it does not work, the electrode should be replaced. The persistence of an artifact after electrode replacement raises the possibility of an artifact from the jackbox connection and the electrode lead pin should be switched with another without an artifact. If the artifact remains in the same channel, it confirms that the jackbox connection is malfunctioning and needs replacement.

4. Use extra electrodes. The appearance of a waveform at the end of the chain electrode can create confusion about cerebral activity versus an extracerebral artifact in the absence of a field. This can be resolved by applying extracerebral electrodes such as supra/infraorbital electrodes for eye movements and electrodes on the cheek for tongue movements. When rhythmic movement artifacts are witnessed (e.g., tremor), applying a pair of surface electrodes over the involved muscle will clarify the origin of the signal.

5. Check the environment and document. Periodic and rhythmic artifacts may be generated by external devices and equipment. Similarly, electrical interference from various devices can generate numerous artifacts. The technologist should carefully look for such equipment, examine the synchrony between the artifact and the generator, and document. When possible and safe, an attempt should be made to eliminate the source of interference and artifact (e.g., switch off the electric bed or mobile phone).

EEG reader

1. Check the impedance. The reader should review the recording settings and look for electrodes with high impedance. This will alert the reader to be on the watch for artifacts involving those electrodes.

2. Re-montage. Using a referential montage reveals the field and facilitates the identification of artifacts confined to a single electrode and non-contiguous field. Be aware of reference contamination, however.

3. Change the filters. Applying the notch filter should eliminate the 50/60 Hz artifact. Elevate the low-frequency filter to remove artifactual slow waves such as a sweat artifact. Similarly, lowering the high-frequency filter setting will reduce high-frequency artifacts. However, be aware of the problem of signal loss and generation of spurious waveforms discussed in a previous chapter. For example, fileting the EMG artifact will leave behind activity resembling beta.

4. Change the timebase. When there are periodic artifacts, compressing the timebase (e.g., from 10 sec/page to 30 sec/page) will highlight the periodicity more clearly.

5. Make use of other polygraphic channels. Other signals such as ECG and EMG channels, whenever available, are useful to correlate with the artifact. Use a vertical cursor to elicit the temporal relationship between the QRS complex of ECG and artifacts seen on the EEG (ECG and pulse artifacts).

6. Review the synchronous video. The modern EEG recordings are almost always accompanied by synchronous video recordings. Reviewing the video will provide very useful information such as movements, the patient touching the electrodes, and other equipment in the vicinity.

7. Read notes made by the technologist. The EEG technologist is on the spot at the time of EEG recording. The observations documented by the EEG technologist are very useful.

References

1. Seneviratne, U. Rational manipulation of digital EEG: Pearls and pitfalls. J Clin Neurophysiol 2014;31:507–516.

2. Beniczky, S, Conradsen, I, Wolf, P. Detection of convulsive seizures using surface electromyography. Epilepsia 2018;59(Suppl 1):23–29.

3. Beniczky, S, Conradsen, I, Moldovan, M, Jennum, P, Fabricius, M, Benedek, K, et al. Quantitative analysis of surface electromyography during epileptic and nonepileptic convulsive seizures. Epilepsia 2014;55:1128–1134.

4. Seneviratne, U, Reutens, D, D'Souza, W. Stereotypy of psychogenic nonepileptic seizures: Insights from video-EEG monitoring. Epilepsia 2010;51:1159–1168.

5. Tyner, FS, Knott, JR, Mayer, WB Jr. Fundamentals of EEG Technology: Volume 1. 1st ed. New York: Raven Press; 1983.

6. Tatum, WO, Dworetzky, BA, Schomer, DL. Artifact and recording concepts in EEG. J Clin Neurophysiol 2011;28:252–263.

CHAPTER 8

Normal variants

There are several electroencephalogram (EEG) patterns that may look abnormal with some resemblance to epileptiform abnormalities and rhythmic bursts. These patterns have been discussed and debated in history, and now there is general agreement that these are normal variants with no clinical significance. It is important to identify normal variants to avoid misinterpretation and misdiagnosis.

Normal variants appear in the form of paroxysmal rhythmic patterns or transients. Pattern recognition plays an important role in the identification of these variants. The reader must pay particular attention to the state of vigilance, location, morphology, amplitude, frequency, duration, rhythmicity, reactivity, and evolution of these patterns. A careful study of the combination of those features will usually make the diagnosis very clear.

RHYTHMIC PATTERNS

Alpha variants

The slow alpha variant is characterized by a subharmonic frequency (half) of the normal alpha rhythm. Similar to the alpha rhythm, the slow alpha variant is biooccipital in distribution and reactive (Figure 8.1a, b & c). It is usually seen admixed with normal alpha rhythm with a sinusoidal or notched morphology.[1] With eye opening and closure, the slow alpha variant behaves exactly like the normal alpha rhythm and it is a good test to identify this variant.

The fast alpha variant has a supraharmonic frequency, usually twice the normal alpha frequency. It is often seen to alternate with the normal alpha rhythm.[1] The distribution and the reactivity are identical to the normal background alpha rhythm.

Posterior slow wave of youth (PSWY)

This pattern is usually seen in young adults (18–30 years). It appears in the posterior head regions admixed with the alpha rhythm and blocked by eye opening and disappears with drowsiness and sleep. It is usually around 3–4 Hz in frequency and alpha activity can often be seen riding on the slow waves. The last alpha wave preceding the ascending limb of the slow wave often appears to dip deeper than other alpha waves below the baseline (Figure 8.2). These slow waves appear randomly or in a semi-rhythmic manner. It may be accentuated by hyperventilation, but photic stimulation has no impact.[2]

The phi rhythm

The phi rhythm (posterior rhythmic slow-wave activity with eye closure) appears within two seconds of eye closure as a run of rhythmic monomorphic bisynchronous delta waves (<4 Hz) over the

DOI: 10.1201/9781003353713-10

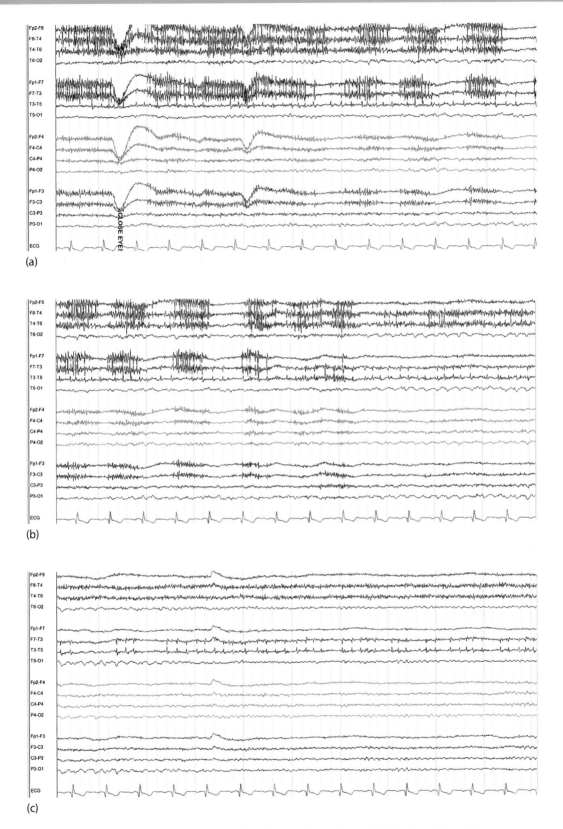

Figure 8.1 Slow alpha variant. (a) Note 10 Hz alpha rhythm in the occipital regions. Slow alpha appears at the end of the epoch. (b) 5 Hz slow alpha activity is seen over the occipital regions. Note the "notched" appearance of the waveform. (c) Reactivity, slow alpha disappears with eye opening.

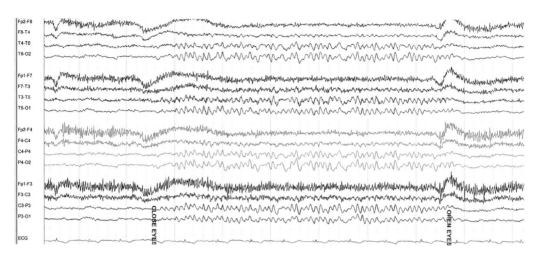

Figure 8.2   Posterior slow wave of youth variant. Note the characteristic morphology and reactivity.

posterior head regions lasting <4 seconds.[3] This rhythm disappears with eye opening. It is usually symmetric with an amplitude twice the alpha rhythm. It is most evident when the subject is alert and with visual attention.[3] This variant starts in childhood (median age 10 years), but may persist into adulthood.[3]

Rhythmic mid-temporal theta of drowsiness (RMTD)

Also known as the psychomotor variant, this pattern is most prevalent in young adults, but can be seen in children and the elderly. As the name implies, rhythmic mid-temporal theta of drowsiness (RMTD) is seen typically in drowsiness over the mid-temporal region in the form of 5–7 Hz rhythmic theta activity.[1] In 10% of subjects, this pattern appears during wakefulness.[4] It has a characteristic sharply-contoured and "notched" appearance. Typically, the maxima are over the mid-temporal regions, however, the field may spread to the parasagittal and occipito-temporal regions. Though typically bilateral and independent, RMTD patterns can be unilateral in 10–27% of subjects.[4,5] The rhythmic trains usually last 1–2 seconds, but occasionally persist for several minutes, creating some doubt about an epileptiform rhythm (Figure 8.3).[4] The lack of evolution is a useful sign to confirm it is not an ictal rhythm (Figure 8.4a–f).

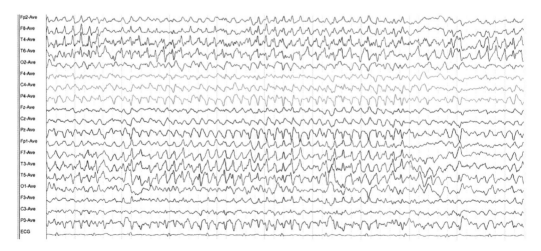

Figure 8.3   Rhythmic mid-temporal theta of drowsiness. This example illustrates a prolonged run of activity with no evolution, which helps to differentiate it from an electrographic seizure. Note the characteristic "notched" appearance of the temporal theta waves.

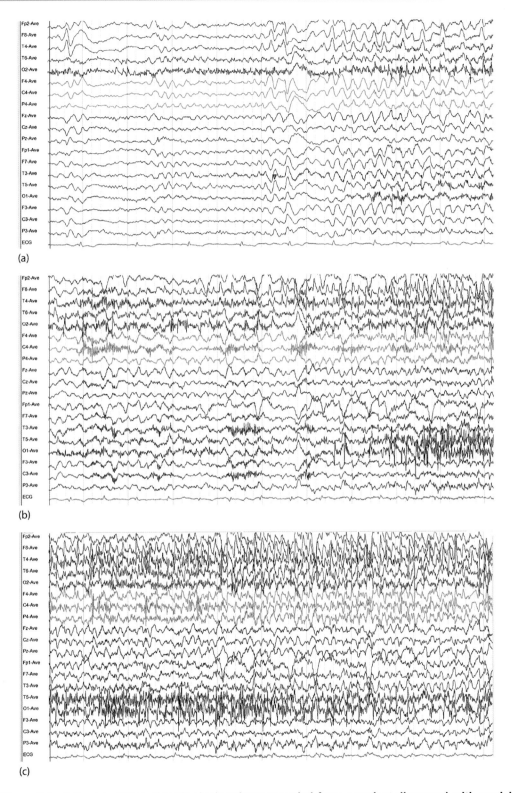

Figure 8.4   A focal to bilateral tonic-clonic seizure recorded from a patient diagnosed with mesial temporal lobe epilepsy with right hippocampal sclerosis. This figure illustrates how the ictal rhythm evolves in comparison with non-evolving rhythmicity in rhythmic mid-temporal theta of drowsiness and subclinical rhythmic electrographic discharges in adults (SREDA). (a) Ictal onset with rhythmic theta activity of right temporal onset, which soon becomes bilateral. Note an interictal sharp- and slow-wave complex

(Continued)

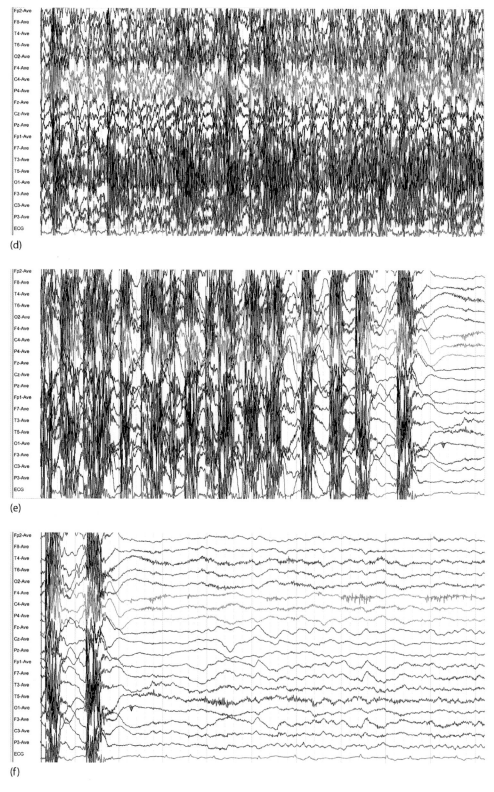

Figure 8.4 *(Continued)* involving F8T4 electrodes at the beginning of the epoch. (b & c) Evolution in frequency. Note the steady increase in the frequency of the right temporal rhythmic activity. The amplitude also increases in parallel. (d) The tonic-clonic phase of the seizure. The ictal rhythm is masked by the muscle and movement artifacts. (e) The terminal part of the seizure with rhythmic clonic activity. (f) Seizure offset and postictal changes. Note the last two clonic jerks followed by postictal suppression and slowing.

Midline theta rhythm of Cigánek

First described by Cigánek in 1961, this pattern appears in the form of trains of 5–7 Hz rhythmic theta activity maximal over the central region (Cz electrode) lasting 4–20 seconds with a waxing and waning appearance.[1,6] However, the field may involve frontal and parasagittal electrodes. Morphologically, it has a spiky and sinusoidal appearance. It is typically seen during wakefulness and drowsiness, while disappearing in sleep.[6] The response to eye opening and other stimuli is variable. This pattern is seen in both children and adults.[6]

Subclinical rhythmic electrographic discharges in adults (SREDA)

Usually seen in people over the age of 50, subclinical rhythmic electrographic discharges in adults (SREDA) is characterized by sharply contoured or sinusoidal monomorphic non-evolving rhythmic theta activity of 5–7 Hz maximal over the parietal and posterior temporal regions lasting from seconds to minutes (Figure 8.5).[7] Comparison of Figure 8.5 with a temporal-lobe seizure pattern (Figure 8.4) highlights the lack of evolution. A SREDA pattern is usually bilateral but can be asymmetric. The onset and offset can be abrupt or gradual. SREDA can be seen during relaxed wakefulness, drowsiness, NREM sleep, hyperventilation, and photic stimulation.[7] The subject remains asymptomatic without any impairment of consciousness or visible signs during SREDA. There is remarkable stereotypy of the pattern on serial recordings of the same subject.[1]

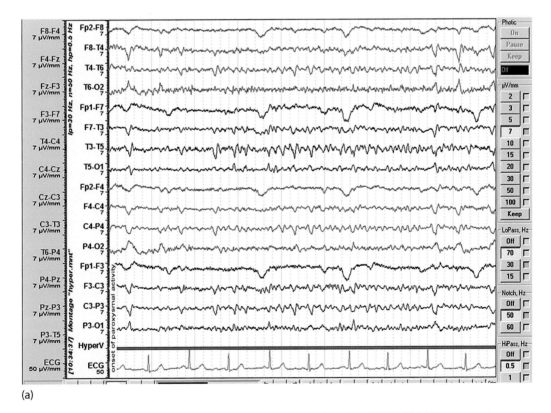

(a)

Figure 8.5 Subclinical rhythmic electrographic discharges in adults (SREDA). (a) The onset of temporal rhythmic theta during hyperventilation. (b & c) Continuation of sharply contoured rhythmic theta without evolution. (d) Abrupt offset without subsequent slowing. *(Continued)*

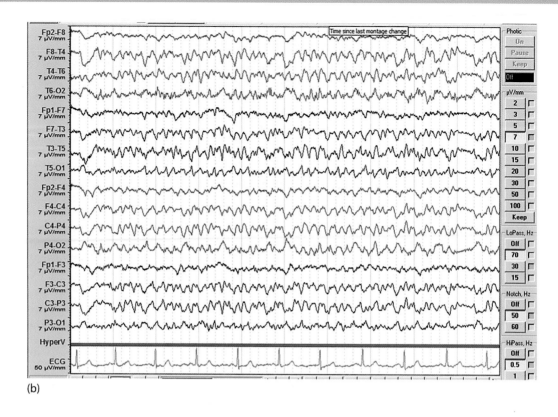

(b)

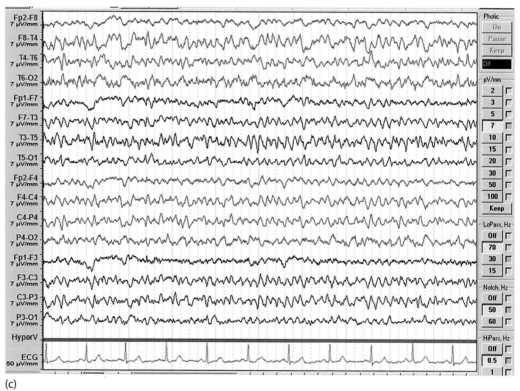

(c)

Figure 8.5 *(Continued)*

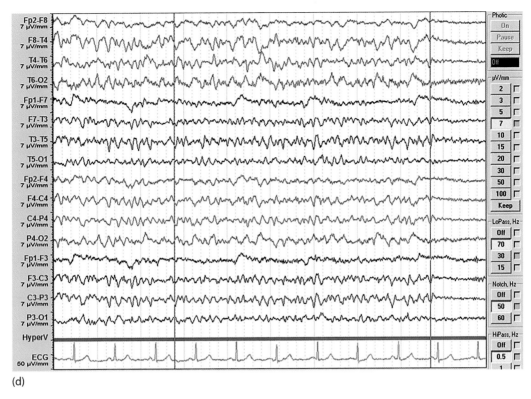

(d)

Figure 8.5 *(Continued)*

Frontal arousal rhythm

Frontal arousal rhythm is seen in children on arousal from sleep and disappears when the child becomes alert. It is characterized by 6.5–8.5 Hz rhythmic activity, predominantly involving F3 and F4 electrodes lasting up to 20 seconds.[8] Harmonics of mixed frequencies give rise to a sharp or notched morphology of the rhythm.[1]

Hypnogogic and hypnopompic hypersynchrony

These patterns are seen in children during drowsiness and arousal. This pattern appears as high-amplitude bursts of generalized 3–4 Hz activity with maxima over the frontocentral regions. This activity can be sustained or paroxysmal.[9] It can be seen in adults under heavy sedation.[10]

TRANSIENTS

14 and 6 Hz positive spike bursts (Ctenoids)

This pattern is seen during drowsiness and light sleep in childhood and adolescence as unilateral or bilateral bursts with shifting predominance and posterior temporal maxima lasting up to 1 second. As the name implies, the bursts consist of surface-positive comb-like spikes occurring at 14 (range 13–17) and/or 6 (range 5–7) Hz.[11] This variant is best visualized on a referential montage (Figure 8.6). Hyperventilation and photic stimulation are effective activation techniques to elicit this variant.[11]

6 Hz spike and wave bursts (phantom spike and wave)

The phantom spike and wave variant is characterized by 5–7 Hz spike-wave bursts lasting up to 1 second with spikes of very low amplitude (<25 microvolts) seen in adults and children. Two distinct subtypes of this variant have been described: WHAM (wake, high amplitude, anterior dominant, male) and FOLD (female, occipital dominant, low amplitude, drowsiness) (Figure 8.7).[12] Both types are benign variants and should not be misdiagnosed as epileptiform abnormalities.

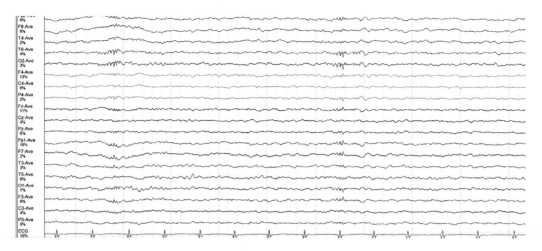

Figure 8.6   14 and 6 Hz positive spike bursts. Note the burst of spikes with positive polarity best visible on T6O2 electrodes.

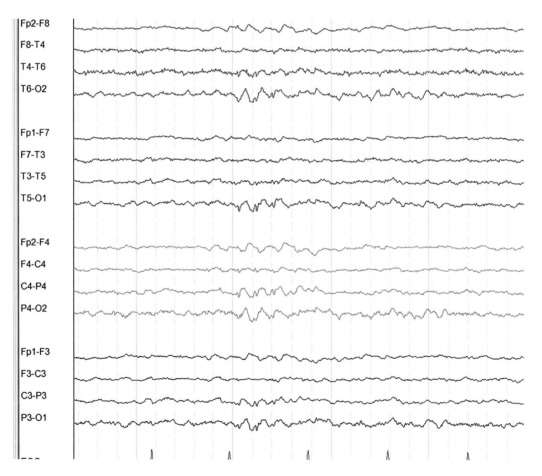

Figure 8.7   6 Hz (phantom) spike and wave bursts. This EEG illustrates the FOLD subtype (female, occipital dominant, low amplitude, drowsiness).

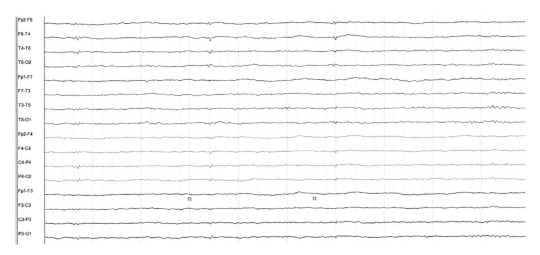

Figure 8.8 Benign sporadic sleep spikes (BSSS). There are three spikes with wide fields visible in this epoch.

Benign sporadic sleep spikes (BSSS)

The benign sporadic sleep spikes (BSSS) variant is also known as small sharp spikes and benign epileptiform transients of sleep. The BSSS pattern is seen during drowsiness and light sleep (stages I and II) and disappearing in slow-wave sleep, usually in adults. Occurring in isolation, the spikes are typically mono- or diphasic with low amplitude (<50 microvolts) and short duration (<50 milliseconds) (Figure 8.8). Occasionally, an after-going slow wave of lower amplitude than spike may be visible. The distribution is unilateral or bilateral (independent or bisynchronous) with temporal maxima.[13]

Wicket spikes

Wicket spikes are seen during drowsiness and light sleep in adults. Morphologically, wickets are monophasic, surface-negative spikes occurring in isolation or trains with a frequency of 6–11 Hz (Figure 8.9).[1] They are usually bilateral and independent with mid-temporal maxima. In contrast to epileptiform spikes, wicket spikes do not disturb the background and are not followed by a slow wave.

Table 8.1 summarizes the key characteristics of all the variants discussed in this chapter.

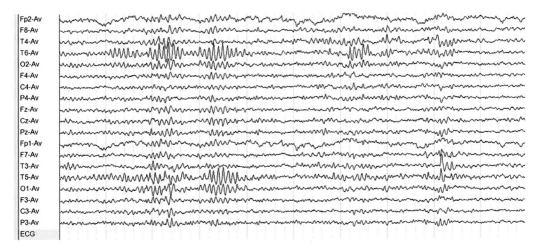

Figure 8.9 Wicket spikes during light sleep involving both temporal regions in this example.

Table 8.1 The summary of key features among normal variants

	Age	State	Distribution	Frequency	Morphology	Duration	Reactivity	Onset and offset	Other features
Slow alpha	Any	Awake	Bioccipital	Half of alpha rhythm	Notched or sinusoidal	Variable	Similar to alpha rhythm	Admixed or alternates with normal alpha rhythm	
Fast alpha	Any	Awake	Bioccipital	Twice the alpha rhythm	Similar to alpha rhythm	Variable	Similar to alpha rhythm	Admixed or alternates with normal alpha rhythm	
PSYW	18–30 y	Awake	Bioccipital	3–4 Hz	Slow wave is a fusion of theta and delta with overriding alpha	Variable	Similar to alpha rhythm	Admixed or alternates with normal alpha rhythm	Accentuated by hyperventilation
Phi rhythm	Children	Awake	Bioccipital	<4 Hz	Monomorphic and bisynchronous	<4 sec	Appears on eye closure, disappears with eye opening	Abrupt onset and offset	Amplitude twice of alpha
RMTD	Young adult	Drowsiness or relaxed wakefulness	Mid-temporal, bilateral, and independent, side-to-side shifting emphasis	4–7 Hz	Sharply contoured with a notch	1–2 sec usually, minutes occasionally	Disappears in deep sleep	Gradual onset and offset	
Cigánek rhythm	Any	Wakefulness and drowsiness	Central with Cz maximum	5–7 Hz	Spiky and sinusoidal	4–20 sec	Disappears in sleep	Waxing and waning	
SREDA	>50 y	Wakefulness, drowsiness, and NREM sleep	Posterior temporal and parietal, unilateral or bilateral asynchronous	5–7 Hz	Sharply contoured or sinusoidal, mono- or biphasic	40–80 seconds	Appears during hyperventilation and photic stimulation	Gradual or abrupt	Recurs multiple times during the same recording, persists on repeated recordings
FAR	Children	Arousal from sleep	Fronto-central F4F3	6–8 Hz	Spindle-like, sharp, notched	<20 sec	Disappears on alertness	Waxing and waning	

(Continued)

Table 8.1 The summary of key features among normal variants *(Continued)*

	Age	State	Distribution	Frequency	Morphology	Duration	Reactivity	Onset and offset	Other features
HHS	children	Drowsiness and arousal	Generalized	3–4 Hz	High amplitude, hypersynchronous, may be notched or spiky	Seconds to minutes	Disappears on alertness	Abrupt onset and offset	
14 & 6 positive spikes	Childhood and adolescence	Drowsiness and light sleep	Posterior temporal maxima, uni- or bilateral	13–17 Hz and 5–7 Hz	Comb-like, positive spikes, amplitude <75 μv	<1 sec	Triggered by hyperventilation and photic stimulation	Abrupt	
Phantom spikes	Children and adults	Wakefulness and drowsiness	Generalized with frontal or occipital maxima	5–7 Hz	Small spike <25 μv, wave <40 μv	<1 sec	Disappears in deep sleep	Abrupt	2 subtypes: WHAM and FOLD
BSSS	Adolescents and adults	Drowsiness and light sleep	Uni or bilateral with temporal maxima		<50 μv amplitude, <50 msec duration, mono- or diphasic		Disappears in slow-wave sleep	Abrupt	
Wicket waves	Adults >30 y	Drowsiness, light sleep, and relaxed wakefulness	Anterior/mid-temporal maxima, unilateral or bilateral independent	6–11 Hz	Trains of monophasic arciform spikes, no slow-wave, 60–200 μv	<1 sec		Abrupt	Shifting predominance, or unilateral predominance

Abbreviations: RMTD = rhythmic mid-temporal theta of drowsiness; SREDA = subclinical rhythmic electrographic discharges in adults; FAR = frontal arousal rhythm; HHS = hypnogogic/hypnopompic hypersynchrony; BSSS = benign sporadic sleep spikes.

References

1. Westmoreland, BF, Klass, DW. Unusual EEG patterns. J Clin Neurophysiol 1990;7:209–228.

2. Aird, RB, Gastaut, Y. Occipital and posterior electroencephalographic rhythms. Electroencephalogr Clin Neurophysiol 1959;11:637–656.

3. Silbert, PL, Radhakrishnan, K, Johnson, J, Klass, DW. The significance of the phi rhythm. Electroencephalogr Clin Neurophysiol 1995;95:71–76.

4. Gibbs, FA, Rich, CL, Gibbs, EL. Psychomotor variant type of seizure discharge. Neurology 1963; 13:991–998.

5. Lipman, IJ, Hughes, JR. Rhythmic mid-temporal discharges. An electro-clinical study. Electroencephalogr Clin Neurophysiol 1969;27:43–47.

6. Westmoreland, BF, Klass, DW. Midline theta rhythm. Arch Neurol 1986;43:139–141.

7. Westmoreland, BF, Klass, DW. A distinctive rhythmic EEG discharge of adults. Electroencephalogr Clin Neurophysiol 1981;51:186–191.

8. White, JC, Tharp, BR. An arousal pattern in children with organic cerebral dysfunction. Electroencephalogr Clin Neurophysiol 1974;37:265–268.

9. Mizrahi, EM. Avoiding the pitfalls of EEG interpretation in childhood epilepsy. Epilepsia 1996; 37:S41–S51.

10. Erwin, CW, Somerville, ER, Radtke, RA. A review of electroencephalographic features of normal sleep. J Clin Neurophysiol 1984;1:253–274.

11. Hughes, JR, Schlagenhauff, RE, Magoss, M. Electro-clinical correlations in the six per second spike and wave complex. Electroencephalogr Clin Neurophysiol 1965;18:71–77.

12. Hughes, JR. Two forms of the 6/sec spike and wave complex. Electroencephalogr Clin Neurophysiol 1980;48:535–550.

13. Tatum, WO, Husain, AM, Benbadis, SR, Kaplan, PW. Normal adult EEG and patterns of uncertain significance. J Clin Neurophysiol 2006;23:194–207.

Abnormal EEG

Clinical applications of EEG in epilepsies and other neurological disorders

CHAPTER 9

The spectrum of epileptiform abnormalities
Interictal, ictal, and ictal-interictal continuum

The distinction between interictal and ictal EEGs can be challenging to the novice. Interictal epileptiform discharges represent "footprints" of epilepsy. It is simply a marker indicating the tendency to generate seizures at some stage. On the contrary, the ictal epileptiform abnormalities indicate a seizure that may be clinical or subclinical. Ictal EEG abnormalities are the definitive signs of seizures. To provide an analogy, if an interictal epileptiform discharge is a spark, the ictal EEG represents the fire.

More recently, it has become apparent that there is a gray zone. These abnormalities are identified as the ictal-interictal continuum. Using the spark and fire analogy, the ictal-interictal continuum can be compared to ember. When the conditions are conducive, these patterns are very likely to become ictal (fire). The ictal-interictal continuum has been described in critically ill patients, usually in the intensive care setting.

INTERICTAL EPILEPTIFORM DISCHARGES

Morphology

Several types of interictal epileptiform discharges have been described based on morphology. Despite variable morphology, all epileptiform discharges have similar clinical significance. The distribution can be focal, multifocal, or generalized depending on the underlying epilepsy syndrome.

1. *Sharp wave:* A waveform with a pointed peak with a duration of 70–200 milliseconds and variable amplitude. The ascending limb is typically steeper than the descending limb, but can be vice versa (Figure 9.1a).[1] Epileptiform sharp waves are usually, but not necessarily, surface-negative.

2. *Sharp and slow-wave complex:* Sharp wave (as described above) followed by a slow wave (Figure 9.1b).

3. *Spike:* A transient with a pointed peak with a duration of 20–70 milliseconds and variable amplitude (usually >50 microvolts) (Figure 9.1c).[1] Similar to sharp waves, the ascending limb is usually steeper than the descending limb and spikes are usually, but not necessarily, surface-negative.

4. *Spike and wave complex:* Spike followed by a surface-negative high-amplitude slow wave (Figure 9.1d).

5. *Polyspikes (polyspike complex):* A sequential run of ≥2 spikes (Figure 9.1e).

6. *Polyspike and wave complex:* Polyspikes followed by a prominent slow wave (Figure 9.1f).

DOI: 10.1201/9781003353713-12

In spike-wave and polyspike-wave complexes, the surface-negative wave is very prominent and of high amplitude often higher than the spike or polyspike. It is not uncommon to see a very small wave after a spike/polyspike, but that does not make it a spike-wave or polyspike-wave complex.

Diagnostic criteria

The main challenge for the EEG reader is to distinguish epileptiform discharges from the background. The reader must be cautious not to overinterpret sharply contoured background activity and normal variants as epileptiform discharges. To confirm a transient as an epileptiform discharge, several criteria must be fulfilled[2]:

1. The discharge is paroxysmal in nature, i.e., the EEG waveform suddenly emerges from the background, reaches the peak rapidly, and then terminates abruptly.

2. The waveform is clearly distinguishable from the background activity with a relatively higher amplitude. It disturbs and stands out from the background.

3. Typically, the epileptiform discharge has a frequency different from the background activity.

4. The waveform has the characteristic morphology of epileptiform discharges as detailed in the previous section.

5. There must be a voltage field with a clear gradient as demonstrated by the involvement of several electrodes (Figure 9.2).

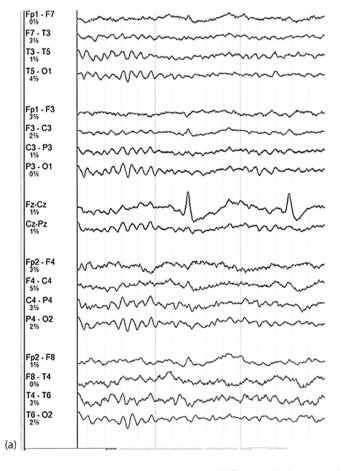

(a)

Figure 9.1   Interictal epileptiform discharges. (a) Sharp wave; (b) Sharp-and-slow wave; (c) Spike; (d) Spike and wave complex. Note that the first discharge is a polyspike and wave complex and the second is a spike and wave complex. (e) Polyspikes; (f) Polyspike and wave complex. Best visible over Fz. *(Continued)*

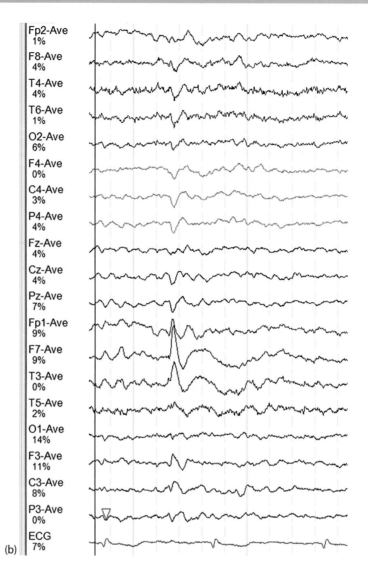

Figure 9.1   *(Continued)*

6. Epileptiform discharges are typically, but not necessarily, surface-negative in polarity.

7. Epileptiform discharges typically have more than one phase. The concept of "phase" has been described in detail in Chapter 4.

More recently, the International Federation of Clinical Neurophysiology has proposed six criteria to identify epileptiform discharges:[1]

1. Waveforms with sharp or spiky morphology and two or three phases.

2. Wave duration is either shorter or longer than the background activity.

3. Ascending and descending components of the sharp wave/spike have different slopes, giving rise to asymmetry.

4. The sharp wave or spike is followed by a slow wave.

5. The discharge disrupts the background activity.

6. Voltage maps reveal a dipole source.

These criteria were validated in a study that found the fulfillment of four or more criteria carried a diagnostic sensitivity of 96%, specificity of 85%, and accuracy of 91%.[3]

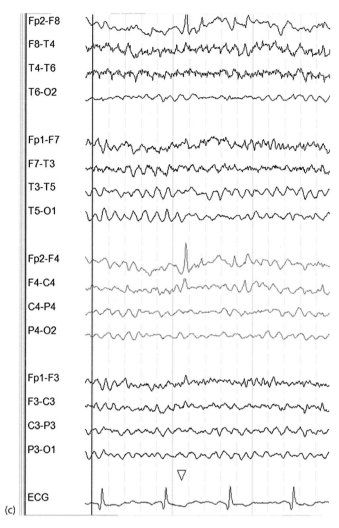

(c)

Figure 9.1   *(Continued)*

Clinical significance

Interictal epileptiform discharges are very useful in clinical practice. However, like any other test, findings should be interpreted in conjunction with clinical details and other investigations. The practical uses include:

1. Confirming the diagnosis of epilepsy.
2. Classification of epilepsy and epilepsy syndromes.
3. Localization of irritative zone in focal epilepsy.
4. Assessment of response to antiepileptic drug therapy and guide antiepileptic drug withdrawal.
5. Providing some guidance on the prognosis.

The diagnostic yield of routine outpatient EEG varies from 10–50% depending on many variables including cohort characteristics and methodological factors.[4] The pre-test probability has a significant impact on the yield, i.e., including patients with a high clinical suspicion of epilepsy will increase the yield. Additionally, the yield can be improved by repeating the test, recording after sleep deprivation, using additional electrodes, use of activations techniques, and increasing the length of recording. Interictal epileptiform discharges are more frequently detected in sleep than

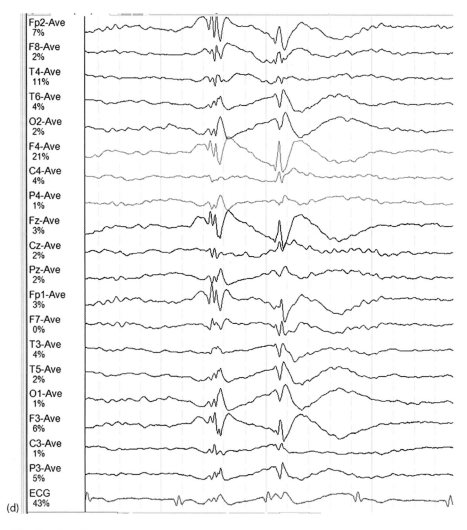

(d)

Figure 9.1 *(Continued)*

in wakefulness.[5] Some antiepileptic drugs tend to decrease the yield.[6] The sensitivity of outpatient EEG to pick up interictal epileptiform discharges is 52%, whereas the specificity is 96%.[7] Hence, it is important to emphasize the fact that epilepsy is a clinical diagnosis supported by investigations including the EEG, and normal EEG does not rule out the diagnosis of epilepsy.

EEG is a vital tool in the classification of epilepsy into generalized, focal, and multifocal depending on the distribution of interictal epileptiform discharges. It is further helpful in identifying epilepsy syndromes. Generalized epileptiform discharges are seen across all idiopathic (genetic) generalized epilepsies, but some characteristics assist in dissecting this large group into several electro-clinical syndromes.[8] The same application is seen in focal epilepsies. For example, benign focal epilepsy in childhood demonstrates characteristic interictal EEG features.[9]

EEG is an indispensable tool in the diagnostic workup for epilepsy surgery. In focal epilepsies, in relation to epilepsy surgery, several overlapping key regions have been identified. This includes the irritative zone, epileptogenic zone, symptomatogenic zone, and functional deficit zone.[10] Interictal epileptiform discharges are conceptualized as representing the irritative zone.[10] It is still very useful in localizing the seizure focus.

Interictal epileptiform discharges may persist with successful antiepileptic drug therapy. The response to therapy is best measured with seizure count as a marker. However, a systematic review

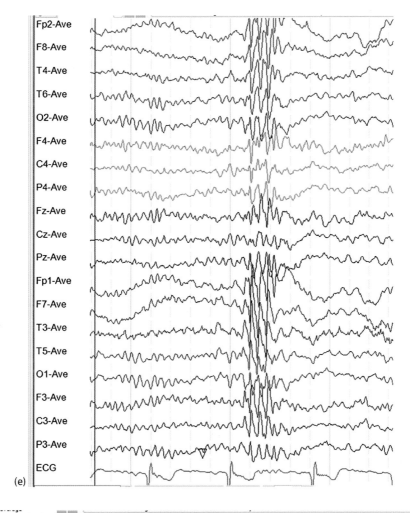

(e)

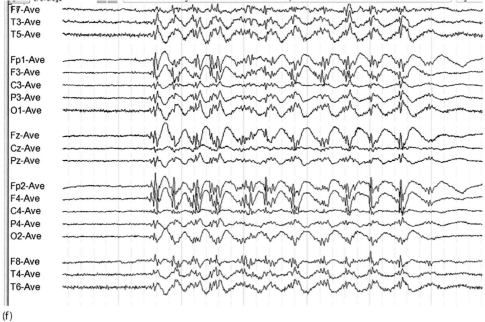

(f)

Figure 9.1   *(Continued)*

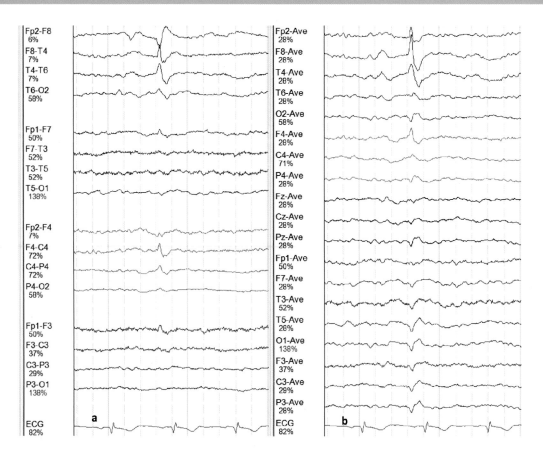

Figure 9.2   Voltage field of an epileptiform discharge. (a) Longitudinal bipolar montage showing a negative phase reversal at the F8 electrode. (b) The voltage field can be clearly visualized on the average reference montage. The sharp wave with the highest amplitude is seen on F8 indicating the "epicenter" of the field. The field spreads to the T4, Fp2, F4, and C4 electrodes. For each discharge, amplitude reduction reflects volume conduction with decreasing amplitude (voltage gradient) that corresponds to the distance away from the voltage maximum of the field.

has reported that in idiopathic generalized epilepsy (IGE), the epileptiform discharge burden tends to be reduced by antiepileptic drug therapy, and that reduction is associated with improved seizure control and cognitive outcomes.[6] Similarly, a meta-analysis found that abnormal EEG with epileptiform discharges predicted a higher rate of seizure relapse following antiepileptic drug withdrawal.[11]

There are several situations where interictal epileptiform discharges provide valuable prognostic information. After the first unprovoked seizure, the presence of epileptiform EEG abnormalities predicts a significantly higher risk of seizure recurrence.[12] In IGE, generalized polyspike train – an interictal EEG abnormality – is a marker of drug resistance.[13] A higher epileptiform discharge burden in IGE is associated with a shorter duration of self-reported seizure freedom.[14] In patients with hippocampal sclerosis who undergo temporal lobectomy, the presence of interictal epileptiform discharges in the post-surgery EEG predicts seizure recurrence upon antiepileptic withdrawal.[15]

Diagnostic pitfalls

Epileptiform discharges have been well documented in people without epilepsy and the prevalence depends on the cohort studied. One study reported epileptiform discharges among 0.5% of healthy aircrew applicants during their medical screening,[16] whereas another study based on referrals to the EEG laboratory reported 12.3%.[17] EEGs of 2.6% of psychiatric inpatients without epilepsy had epileptiform discharges in a study.[18] Antipsychotic drugs may have played a role there. A meta-analysis found that clozapine significantly increases the risk of epileptiform EEG abnormalities among psychiatric patients without epilepsy (odds ratio = 17).[19] Another important factor to consider is a family history of epilepsy. One study reported epileptiform EEG abnormalities among 6% of asymptomatic first-degree relatives of probands with juvenile myoclonic epilepsy.[20]

There are several normal variants that can be misdiagnosed as epileptiform discharges due to close morphological resemblance. These variants include rhythmic mid temporal theta of drowsiness, wicket spikes, phantom spike and wave, and benign sporadic sleep spikes as detailed in Chapter 8. Overinterpretation of normal variants leads to misdiagnosis of epilepsy.[21]

Misclassification of epilepsy is not uncommon. Generalized epilepsy may be misclassified as focal epilepsy due to the presence of focal and asymmetric epileptiform discharges. Similarly, focal epilepsy can be misdiagnosed as generalized epilepsy due to secondary bilateral synchrony, particularly in frontal lobe epilepsy. The phenomenon of "secondary bilateral synchrony" will be explained in detail in Chapter 10.

The diagnostic pitfall caused by false lateralization of midline foci has been described in Chapter 3 (Figure 9.3a & b). Patients with large cerebral lesions causing seizures may also show false lateralization of epileptiform discharges on the contralateral hemisphere with the surface EEG.[22,23]

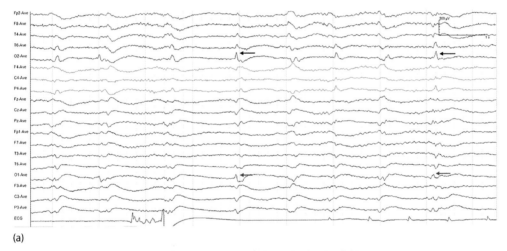

(a)

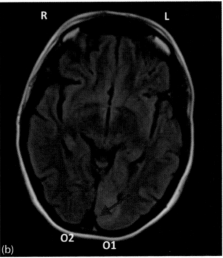

(b)

Figure 9.3 Paradoxical lateralization of interictal epileptiform discharges. (a) Sharp waves are seen over O2 (black arrows) and O1 (red arrows) electrodes with a higher amplitude over O2, suggesting a midline occipital focus closer to O2. (b) The MRI brain scan shows a lesion in the left mesial occipital region. Even though the epileptogenic lesion is on the left, the right occipital electrode has the best "view," so records a higher amplitude.

ICTAL EPILEPTIFORM ABNORMALITIES

EEG seizure patterns we observe depend on the underlying epileptic networks. Ictal rhythms of generalized epilepsies, focal epilepsies, and epileptic encephalopathies will be described in detail in subsequent chapters. In this chapter, we will discuss some general principles.

Rhythmicity is the key feature in an ictal rhythm. On the surface EEG, four main EEG seizure patterns can be identified: repetitive spikes or spike-wave discharges, electrodecremental pattern, generalized paroxysmal fast activity, and evolving ictal rhythms. The onset of the ictal rhythm indicates the seizure onset zone. In generalized epilepsies, the onset of the ictal rhythm is generalized, i.e., involving all electrodes bilaterally at the same timepoint. Typically, in focal epilepsies, the onset is seen over a limited number of electrodes before spatiotemporal evolution. For example, in a left mesial temporal seizure, the ictal onset is seen over F7T3 electrodes. When the onset is not well-localized on the surface EEG but confined to a single hemisphere, it is called "lateralized onset." There are occasions where the onset is unclear due to artifacts.

Non-evolving and monomorphic repetitive spiking/spike-wave discharges

This pattern is usually seen in generalized epilepsies (Figure 9.4). If the EEG pattern is accompanied by a clinical seizure, it is easy to diagnose as a seizure pattern regardless of the duration of the event. The challenge is differentiating interictal from ictal when the clinical features are not evident or documented. An arbitrary time limit of ≥3 seconds is often used in absence seizures of generalized epilepsies to define an ictal rhythm with repetitive spiking. In critical care EEG, a run of epileptiform discharges with >2.5 Hz frequency continuing for 10 or more seconds is considered an electrographic seizure.

Diffuse electrodecremental pattern

The diffuse electrodecremental pattern as an ictal rhythm appears in two forms: (a) generalized low-voltage (<25 microvolts) fast activity (>15 Hz) or (b) generalized attenuation of EEG activity without an overriding fast component (Figure 9.5).[24] This ictal rhythm has been described in association with tonic and atonic seizures, usually in the setting of epileptic encephalopathies.[24,25] There is no time criterion to define a diffuse electrodecremental pattern and it usually is brief, lasting <10 seconds.

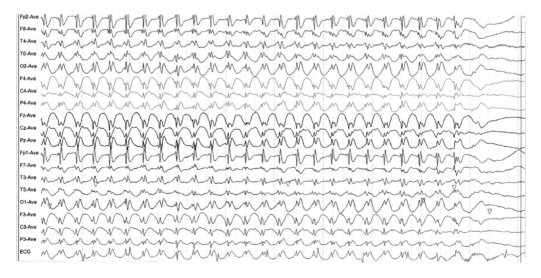

Figure 9.4   Repetitive spiking as an ictal rhythm as illustrated by an absence seizure.

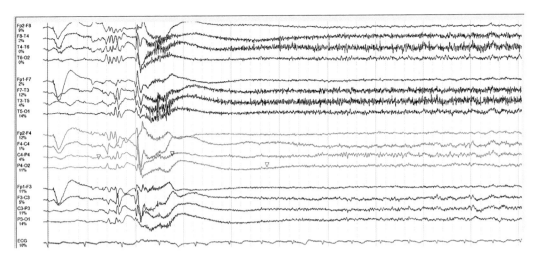

Figure 9.5   Electrodecremental pattern of a tonic seizure in Lennox-Gastaut syndrome.

Generalized paroxysmal fast activity

Typically described in association with tonic seizures in Lennox-Gastaut syndrome, the generalized paroxysmal fast activity (GPFA) has also been observed in other epileptic encephalopathies, focal epilepsies, and generalized epilepsies. Electrographically, GPFA is characterized by generalized paroxysms of high-amplitude (100–200 microvolts), high-frequency (8–25 Hz) rhythmic spike discharges of frontocentral dominance lasting ≥1 second, most frequently appearing in NREM sleep (see Chapter 12 for an example).[26–29] Though typically generalized, amplitude asymmetries are observed in some cases of GPFA.[29] The distinction between ictal and interictal GPFA is difficult. Tonic seizure activity is the semiological hallmark of GPFA. However, the ictal semiological features associated with GPFA can be quite subtle, such as eye opening, eyelid flutter, head version, eye deviation, jaw opening, and changes in breathing.[26,28] Paroxysms tend to be longer during wakefulness (mean 6 seconds versus 3 seconds in sleep) and more frequently associated with clinically obvious seizure manifestations (100% versus 47% in sleep).[26] Studies have demonstrated subclinical tonic activity on electromyography channels during GPFA without visible clinical semiology.[30] Hence, for all practical purposes, GPFA can be considered an ictal rhythm with a varying degree of semiological manifestations ranging from subclinical to overtly clinical.

Evolving ictal rhythm

This ictal pattern is seen in seizures of focal onset. There are two key elements in this seizure pattern: seizure onset and evolution. The identification of electrographic seizure onset is often a challenge. It is characterized by a change in the background, but can be subtle at times. There are five EEG patterns that mark the ictal onset[31]:

1. Focal spikes or sharp waves.
2. Rhythmic activity of any frequency.
3. Attenuation of the background activity.
4. Baseline direct current shifts/infraslow activity.
5. High frequency oscillations.

Following the onset, the ictal rhythm must evolve. Morphologically, the ictal rhythm may consist of epileptiform discharges, rhythmic frequencies (alpha, beta, theta, delta, gamma), or a mix of both. Evolution means a sequential change in one or more of the three characteristics: frequency, morphology, and location. Changes in amplitude are also very useful and easy to visualize with an evolving seizure pattern (Figure 9.6a & b). The duration of evolution needed to diagnose an

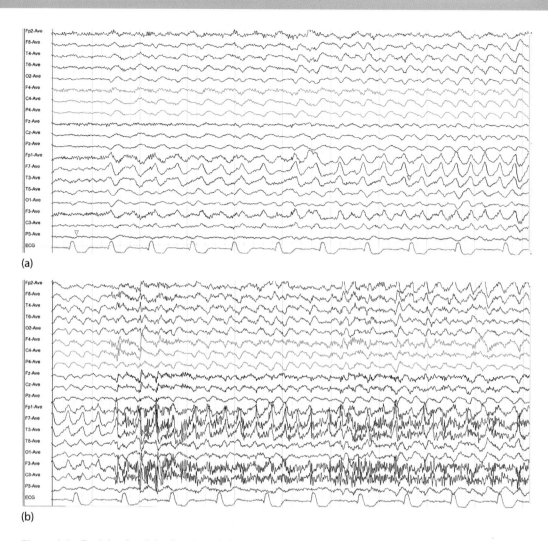

(a)

(b)

Figure 9.6   Evolving ictal rhythm. (a) Left frontotemporal ictal onset (F7T3). Note that 2 Hz rhythmic activity at the onset becomes 3 Hz toward the end of the epoch. The morphology also changes with increasing amplitude. (b) A further increase in the frequency of the rhythmic activity to 4 Hz with changing morphology. Note the gradual spread of the activity to other electrodes from the onset.

electrographic seizure is somewhat arbitrary. In critical care EEG terminology, an evolving rhythm lasting for 10 or more seconds is defined as an electrographic seizure whereas an evolving pattern of <10 seconds is called 'brief potentially ictal rhythmic discharges-BIRDs' (see Chapter 15).

Evolution in frequency

According to the American Clinical Neurophysiology Society criteria, evolution in frequency is defined as two or more consecutive increases or decreases in frequency by ≥0.5 Hz in the same direction with each change persisting for three or more cycles.[32] Additionally, each change should last <5 minutes.[32] For example, the frequency changes can be 2 Hz–>2.5 Hz–>3 Hz or 3 Hz–>2 Hz–>1.5 Hz. Each change must last at least three cycles. For example, 3 Hz must last ≥1 second and 1.5 Hz must last ≥2 seconds.

Evolution in location

The evolution in location is defined as sequentially involving two or more different electrodes with each change persisting for three or more cycles. Additionally, each change should last <5 minutes. For example, a 3 Hz rhythmic activity appears in T4, spreading to T6 persisting for ≥1 second, followed by the involvement of C4 lasting for ≥1 second.

Evolution in morphology

The evolution in morphology is defined as sequentially changing to two or more novel morphologies with each change persisting for three or more cycles. Additionally, each change should last <5 minutes.

Diagnostic pitfalls

Similar to interictal discharges, ictal onset on the surface EEG can show false lateralization to the contralateral hemisphere in cases of midline foci and large cerebral lesions.[22,23,33] Surface EEG may not pick up the ictal rhythm if the involved region is small or deep. Only 21% of simple focal seizures were found to be accompanied by visible changes on the surface EEG in a study.[34] Additionally, muscle and movement artifacts can completely mask the underlying EEG ictal rhythm. Hence, care should be exercised in excluding seizures in a symptomatic patient without a demonstrable ictal rhythm.

ICTAL-INTERICTAL CONTINUUM

The ictal-interictal continuum has been proposed as the border zone between the ictal and interictal/encephalopathy spectrum of EEG rhythms in critically ill patients.[35] This group includes several rhythmic and periodic patterns, such as lateralized periodic discharges, generalized periodic discharges, bilateral independent periodic discharges, lateralized rhythmic delta activity, and generalized rhythmic delta activity. Differentiating these patterns from pure encephalopathic patterns poses a challenge. The ictal-interictal continuum will be discussed in detail under the critical care EEG section (Chapter 15).

References

1. Kane, N, Acharya, J, Benickzy, S, et al. A revised glossary of terms most commonly used by clinical electroencephalographers and updated proposal for the report format of the EEG findings. Revision 2017. Clin Neurophysiol Pract 2017;2:170–185.

2. Pillai, J, Sperling, MR. Interictal EEG and the diagnosis of epilepsy. Epilepsia 2006;47(Suppl 1):14–22.

3. Kural, MA, Duez, L, Sejer Hansen, V, et al. Criteria for defining interictal epileptiform discharges in EEG. A clinical validation study. Neurology 2020;94:e2139–e2147.

4. Monif, M, Seneviratne, U. Clinical factors associated with the yield of routine outpatient scalp electroencephalograms: A retrospective analysis from a tertiary hospital. J Clin Neurosci 2017;45:110–114.

5. Seneviratne, U, Boston, RC, Cook, M, D'Souza, W. Temporal patterns of epileptiform discharges in genetic generalized epilepsies. Epilepsy Behav 2016;64:18–25.

6. Gunawan, C, Seneviratne, U, D'Souza, W. The effect of antiepileptic drugs on epileptiform discharges in genetic generalized epilepsy: A systematic review. Epilepsy Behav 2019;96:175–182.

7. Goodin, DS, Aminoff, MJ. Does the interictal EEG have a role in the diagnosis of epilepsy? Lancet 1984;1:837–839.

8. Seneviratne, U, Hepworth, G, Cook, M, D'Souza, W. Can EEG differentiate among syndromes in genetic generalized epilepsy? J Clin Neurophysiol 2017;34:213–221.

9. Pan, A, Lüders, HO. Epileptiform discharges in benign focal epilepsy of childhood. Epileptic Disord 2000;2(Suppl 1):S29–36.

10. Nair, DR, Burgess, MA, Luders, R. A critical review of the different conceptual hypotheses framing human focal epilepsy. Epileptic Disord 2004;6:77–83.

11. Berg, AT, Shinnar, S. Relapse following discontinuation of antiepileptic drugs: A meta-analysis. Neurology 1994;44:601–608.

12. Berg, AT, Shinnar, S. The risk of seizure recurrence following A first unprovoked seizure: A quantitative review. Neurology 1991;41:965–972.

13. Sun, Y, Seneviratne, U, Perucca, P, et al. Generalized polyspike train: An EEG biomarker of drug-resistant idiopathic generalized epilepsy. Neurology 2018;91:e1822–e1830.

14. Seneviratne, U, Boston, RC, Cook, M, D'Souza, W. EEG correlates of seizure freedom in genetic generalized epilepsies. Neurol Clin Pract 2017;7:35–44.

15. Rathore, C, Sarma, SP, Radhakrishnan, K. Prognostic importance of serial postoperative EEGs after anterior temporal lobectomy. Neurology 2011;76:1925–1931.

16. Gregory, RP, Oates, T, Merry, RT. Electroencephalogram epileptiform abnormalities in candidates for aircrew training. Electroencephalogr Clin Neurophysiol 1993;86:75–77.

17. Sam, MC, So, EL. Significance of epileptiform discharges in patients without epilepsy in the community. Epilepsia 2001;42:1273–1278.

18. Bridgers, SL. Epileptiform abnormalities discovered on electroencephalographic screening of psychiatric inpatients. Arch Neurol 1987;44:312–316.

19. Jackson, A, Seneviratne, U. EEG changes in patients on antipsychotic therapy: A systematic review. Epilepsy Behav 2019;95:1–9.

20. Jayalakshmi, SS, Mohandas, S, Sailaja, S, Borgohain, R. Clinical and electroencephalographic study of first-degree relatives and probands with juvenile myoclonic epilepsy. Seizure 2006;15:177–183.

21. Benbadis, SR, Lin, K. Errors in EEG interpretation and misdiagnosis of epilepsy. Which EEG patterns are overread? Eur Neurol 2008;59:267–271.

22. Sammaritano, M, de Lotbinière, A, Andermann, F, Olivier, A, Gloor, P, Quesney, LF. False lateralization by surface EEG of seizure onset in patients with temporal lobe epilepsy and gross focal cerebral lesions. Ann Neurol 1987;21:361–369.

23. Teixeira, RA, Li, LM, Santos, SLM, et al. Laterization of epileptiform discharges in patients with epilepsy and precocious destructive brain insults. Arq Neuropsiquiatr 2004;62:1–8.

24. Arroyo, S, Lesser, RP, Fisher, RS, et al. Clinical and electroencephalographic evidence for sites of origin of seizures with diffuse electrodecremental pattern. Epilepsia 1994;35:974–987.

25. Fariello, RG, Doro, JM, Forster, FM. Generalized cortical electrodecremental event. Clinical and neurophysiological observations in patients with dystonic seizures. Arch Neurol 1979;36:285–291.

26. Brenner, RP, Atkinson, R. Generalized paroxysmal fast activity: Electroencephalographic and clinical features. Ann Neurol 1982;11:386–390.

27. Halasz, P, Janszky, J, Barcs, G, Szucs, A. Generalised paroxysmal fast activity (GPFA) is not always a sign of malignant epileptic encephalopathy. Seizure 2004;13:270–276.

28. Markand, ON. Lennox-Gastaut syndrome (childhood epileptic encephalopathy). J Clin Neurophysiol 2003;20:426–441.

29. Mohammadi, M, Okanishi, T, Okanari, K, et al. Asymmetrical generalized paroxysmal fast activities in children with intractable localization-related epilepsy. Brain Dev 2015;37:59–65.

30. Chatrian, GE, Lettich, E, Wilkus, RJ, Vallarta, J. Polygraphic and clinical observations on tonic-autonomic seizures. Electroencephalogr Clin Neurophysiol Suppl 1982:101–124.

31. Rodin, E, Constantino, T, Rampp, S, Modur, P. Seizure onset determination. J Clin Neurophysiol 2009;26:1–12.

32. Hirsch, LJ, LaRoche, SM, Gaspard, N, et al. American Clinical Neurophysiology Society's Standardized Critical Care EEG Terminology: 2012 version. J Clin Neurophysiol 2013;30:1–27.

33. Catarino, CB, Vollmar, C, Noachtar, S. Paradoxical lateralization of non-invasive electroencephalographic ictal patterns in extra-temporal epilepsies. Epilepsy Res 2012;99:147–155.

34. Devinsky, O, Kelley, K, Porter, RJ, Theodore, WH. Clinical and electroencephalographic features of simple partial seizures. Neurology 1988;38:1347–1347.

35. Chong, DJ, Hirsch, LJ. Which EEG patterns warrant treatment in the critically ill? Reviewing the evidence for treatment of periodic epileptiform discharges and related patterns. J Clin Neurophysiol 2005;22:79–91.

CHAPTER 10

EEG of genetic generalized epilepsies

Genetic generalized epilepsy (GGE) encompasses several electroclinical syndromes diagnosed and classified according to clinical features and electroencephalogram (EEG) characteristics.[1-3] The EEG hallmark of GGE is bilateral synchronous, symmetrical, and generalized spike-wave (GSW) discharges. Polyspikes and polyspike-wave discharges are also commonly seen in GGE. Fixation-off sensitivity (FOS), eye-closure sensitivity, photoparoxysmal response, epileptiform K-complexes/sleep spindles, and occipital intermittent rhythmic delta activity (OIRDA) are among the spectrum of abnormalities described in GGE.[4]

INTERICTAL VERSUS ICTAL ABNORMALITIES

Interictal EEG abnormalities are defined as "epileptiform patterns occurring singly or in bursts lasting at most a few seconds," whereas ictal rhythms consist of "repetitive EEG discharges with a relatively abrupt onset and termination and characteristic pattern of evolution lasting at least several seconds."[5] Subclinical seizure activity refers to EEG seizure patterns not accompanied by clinical signs and symptoms.[5] However, in absence seizures, differentiating interictal from ictal epileptiform discharges can be difficult as those discharges demonstrate monomorphic rhythmicity with little evolution. Consequently, the distinction between ictal and interictal activity depends on how long it lasts and clinical features, particularly impairment of consciousness during the discharge. Researchers have used several testing methods, including reaction time and motor tasks to study cognition and the degree of consciousness during spike-wave discharges.[6]

There is no consensus on the duration of the GSW paroxysm that defines an absence seizure. Some researchers have defined absence seizures based on two criteria: (1) generalized spike-wave activity of any duration when accompanied by clinical signs, and (2) GSW lasting >2 seconds even if not accompanied by clinical correlates. Discharges of <2 seconds in duration without clinical signs were identified as interictal fragments.[7] Another study considered GSW bursts lasting ≥3 seconds, with or without clinical signs, as an absence seizure.[8]

Conversely, myoclonic seizures and generalized tonic-clonic seizures (GTCS) demonstrate well-characterized EEG changes and the distinction from interictal EEG abnormalities is clearly defined.[4]

INTERICTAL ABNORMALITIES

Spike-wave complex

Morphology and amplitude

Gibbs et al. published the first detailed analysis of the spike-wave complex.[9,10] Subsequently, a more detailed analysis has revealed three components of the spike (spike 1, positive transient, and spike 2).[11] The surface-negative spike 1 is of low amplitude (25–50 microvolt) and brief duration (10 milliseconds).

DOI: 10.1201/9781003353713-13

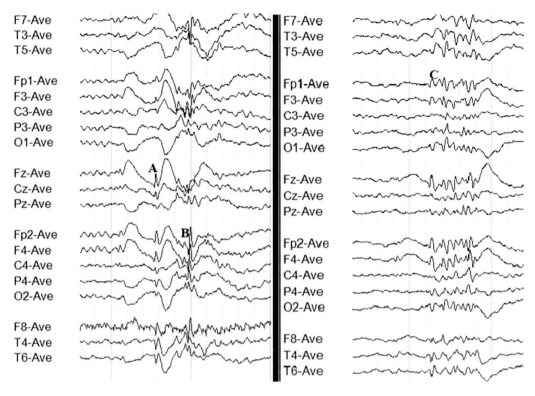

Figure 10.1 Typical interictal epileptiform discharges in genetic generalized epilepsy. Note the bilateral, symmetrical, and synchronous spike-wave discharges (a), polyspike-wave discharges (b), and polyspikes (c).

The second component is a positive transient of 100–150 milliseconds. It is followed by spike 2 of negative polarity lasting 30–60 milliseconds with frontal amplitude maxima. The dome-shaped wave of negative polarity, which follows the spike, lasts 150–200 milliseconds (Figure 10.1).[11] However, spike 1 is seen less consistently than spike 2.[12]

A study based on 24-hour ambulatory EEGs found 96.4% of generalized epileptiform discharges to be symmetric. However, the typical morphology was observed in only 24%.[13]

Topography

Typically, the maximum amplitude is seen over the frontocentral region. With the use of three-dimensional (3-D) field potential maps, researchers were able to demonstrate that the amplitude maximum of spikes was over the frontal region involving anterior and midline electrodes.[14] Using quantitative EEG analysis, researchers were able to demonstrate increased activity over the prefrontal region in patients diagnosed with GGE.[15] The field maxima during absence seizures are usually detected at the Fz electrode with lateral spread to F3 and F4, and posterior spread to Cz electrode.[16] The amplitude maximum of the spike-wave complex is most frequently observed in the frontocentral region (96.3%), followed by frontopolar (2.4%) and occipital (1.3%) regions.[13]

Further insights into topography have been revealed in studies using quantitative EEG techniques. The source localization of epileptiform discharges on dense array EEG in juvenile myoclonic epilepsy (JME) detected activity in the orbitofrontal and medial frontopolar cortex.[17] Another study using three techniques of source imaging analysis found the anterior cingulate cortex and medial frontal gyrus as the primary anatomical sources of generalized spike-wave discharges in GGE.[18]

Regularity

In EEG, regularity refers to waveforms with relatively uniform morphology.[5] The classic electrographic feature in GGE is regular and rhythmic generalized spike-wave discharges. Nonetheless, a recent study has reported that 60% of generalized spike-wave paroxysms are irregular.[13]

Frequency of discharges

The typical 3 Hz spike-wave activity characteristic of absence seizures was first described by Gibbs and collaborators.[9] The fast spike-wave activity of >3.5 Hz is usually seen in JME.[19] The spike-wave discharge frequency in juvenile absence epilepsy (JAE) (mean 3.25 Hz) is faster than childhood absence epilepsy (CAE) and slower than JME.[7] In spike-wave paroxysms, the frequency is not constant throughout. The initial frequency is slightly faster and then it becomes more stable, slower, and regular.[20]

Background

Typically, epileptiform discharges emerge from a normal background in GGE.[2] Generalized epileptiform discharges occurring on a slow and disorganized background raise the possibility of an epileptic encephalopathy.[21,22]

Polyspikes and polyspike-wave discharges

Polyspikes are characterized by a run of two or more spikes, whereas the polyspike-wave complex consists of polyspikes followed by slow waves.[5] In GGE, polyspikes usually occur in the form of high-amplitude rhythmic bursts with synchronized and generalized distribution (Figure 10.1).

Photoparoxysmal response

This is an abnormal response manifesting with the generation of spike-wave complexes, polyspikes, or polyspike-wave discharges during intermittent photic stimulation.[5] The photoparoxysmal response (PPR) is under the influence of several confounding variables including age, sex, ethnicity, genetics, antiepileptic medication use, state of alertness (sleep versus wakefulness), sleep deprivation, and the stimulation technique. There are three grades of PPR: (1) posterior stimulus-dependent response, (2) posterior stimulus-independent response, and (3) generalized response.[23] The response to photic stimulation is defined as self-sustained when the epileptiform discharges outlast the stimulus by ≥100 milliseconds.[24] PPR is most frequently detected in juvenile myoclonic epilepsy (83%) followed by childhood absence epilepsy (21%) and JAE (25%).[7] However, PPR can also be elicited in 0.3 to 4% of adults without a history of epilepsy.[25,26] It is detected more frequently (14.2%) in asymptomatic children.[27] The influence of various confounders including stimulation techniques may explain the wide range of results reported in the literature.

Eye-closure sensitivity

Epileptiform discharges characteristic of eye-closure sensitivity emerge within 1–3 seconds of eye closure and last for 1–4 seconds. However, the discharges do not persist for the total duration when the eyes remain closed (Figure 10.2). Photosensitivity and eye-closure sensitivity are related phenomena.[28]

Fixation-off sensitivity

Epileptiform discharges, generalized or occipital, triggered by the elimination of fixation and central vision are the hallmarks of FOS.[29] This abnormality needs to be distinguished from photosensitivity and eye-closure sensitivity. In FOS, epileptiform discharges persist for the total duration of eye closure and disappear on eye opening (Figure 10.2).[29] To confirm FOS, central vision and fixation should be eliminated with the application of spherical lenses, Frenzel lenses, or Ganzfeld stimulation technique.[30] FOS has been described in GGE and occipital epilepsy.[30] In some patients, photosensitivity and FOS may coexist.[31]

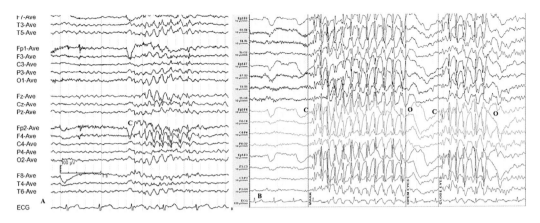

Figure 10.2 Eye-closure sensitivity and fixation-off sensitivity in genetic generalized epilepsy. (a) Generalized spike-wave and polyspike-wave discharges appear after eye closure (C) and fade away after one second indicating eye-closure sensitivity. (b) Generalized epileptiform discharges appear with eye closure (C), continue as long as eyes are closed, and disappear on eye opening (O), indicating fixation-off sensitivity.

Epileptiform K-complexes and sleep spindles

The overlap between generalized epileptiform discharges and K-complexes (epileptiform K-complexes) as well as sleep spindles (epileptiform sleep spindles) has been described.[32,33] This overlap generates complexes with very characteristic morphology and topography (Figure 10.3).[33] A recent study has found this to be common in GGE with 65% of patients demonstrating epileptiform K-complexes and 10% epileptiform sleep spindles.[34] These abnormalities probably indicate the link between microarousals and epileptiform discharges in GGE.[34]

Occipital intermittent rhythmic delta activity

OIRDA is characterized by transient unilateral or bilateral occipital runs of 2–3 Hz, regular, rhythmic, and sinusoidal delta activity.[5] Deep stages of sleep and eye opening typically attenuate OIRDA, whereas drowsiness and hyperventilation make it more prominent (Figure 10.4a & b).[35] It is detected in approximately one-third of patients diagnosed with CAE.[36] Though often reported as an EEG abnormality of CAE, OIRDA is not specific to epilepsy and can be seen in encephalopathies, particularly in children.[35]

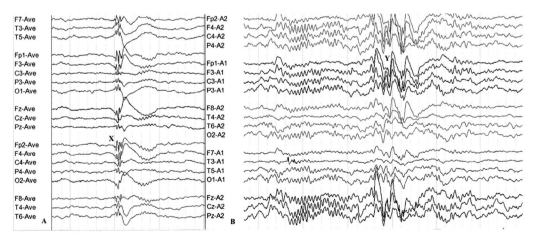

Figure 10.3 Epileptiform K-complexes and sleep spindles in genetic generalized epilepsy. (a) Polyspikes overlap with a K-complex at X. (b) A burst of generalized spike-wave discharges (Y) in the midst of a sleep spindle.

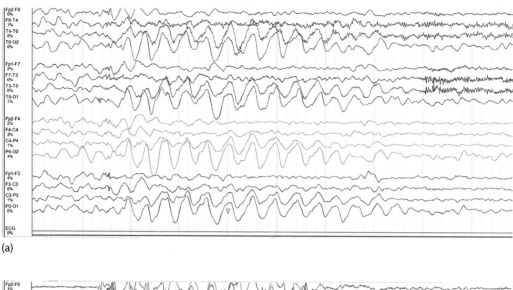

(a)

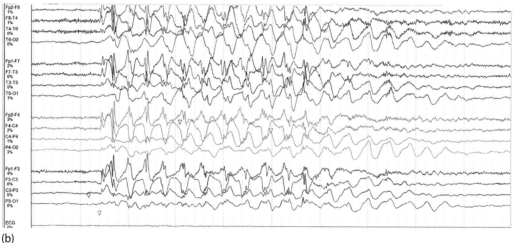

(b)

Figure 10.4 Occipital intermittent rhythmic delta activity. (a) Occipital intermittent rhythmic delta activity during hyperventilation in a child diagnosed with childhood absence epilepsy. (b) An absence seizure captured during the same EEG recording. Note the terminal part of the seizure resembles OIRDA.

ICTAL EEG CHANGES

Myoclonic seizures

High-amplitude, generalized, polyspike activity of 10–16 Hz with the frontocentral maximum is the EEG hallmark of myoclonic seizures.[19,37] These typical discharges may be preceded by irregular 2–5 Hz GSW activity and sometimes followed by irregular slow waves of 1–3 Hz (Figure 10.5).[19,37,38] The EEG seizure may be several seconds longer than the clinical seizure.[37,38]

Typical absence seizures

Bilateral, regular, symmetrical, and synchronous 3 Hz spike-wave activity (range 2.5–4 Hz) sometimes admixed with polyspike-wave discharges on a normal background is the hallmark of a typical absence seizure (Figure 10.6).[39,40] There are some differences among syndromes.

It is not unusual for the initial ictal discharge to be atypical. It could be non-generalized, spike-wave, polyspike-wave, or irregular discharges, with typical GSW activity appearing after an average of 0.7 seconds.[7]

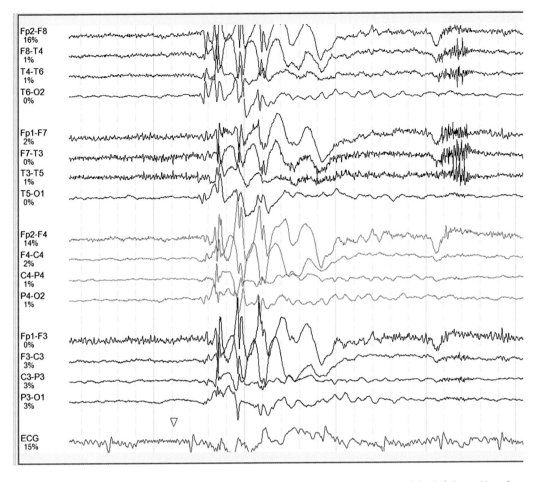

Figure 10.5   EEG of a myoclonic seizure. A burst of generalized polyspike-wave activity is followed by a few slow waves.

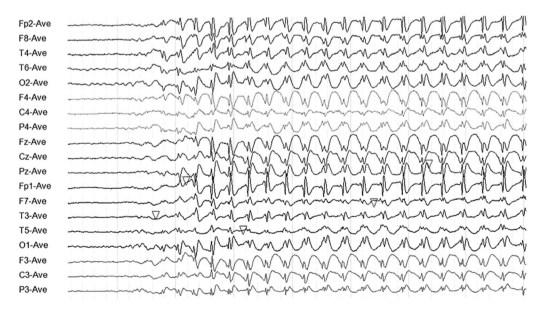

Figure 10.6   EEG of a typical absence seizure. Note the paroxysm of generalized, symmetrical, synchronous, and regular 3 Hz spike-wave discharges of frontocentral maxima.

Myoclonic absence seizures

Myoclonic absence seizures are semiologically characterized by absences in association with tonic contractions, resulting in progressive upper-limb elevation and superimposed rhythmic myoclonic jerks.[2] The impairment of awareness is less pronounced in comparison to typical absence seizures. Both myoclonic absence and typical absence seizure have similar ictal EEG patterns (Figure 10.7).[2,41] Polygraphic recordings are useful to demonstrate the correlation between the ictal EEG and tonic as well as myoclonic activity. Often triggered by hyperventilation, myoclonic absence seizures are less frequently (14%) induced by intermittent photic stimulation.[41]

Absence seizures with eyelid myoclonia

Eyelid myoclonia with absences, EEG paroxysms/seizures triggered by eye closure, and photosensitivity are the main features of Jeavons syndrome.[42] Sometimes, eyelid myoclonia may not be associated with an absence seizure.[42] The ictal EEG typically shows generalized high-amplitude polyspikes and polyspike-wave discharges of 3–6 Hz lasting 1.5 to 6 seconds (Figure 10.8).[42] The ictal discharges occur with or before the onset of eyelid myoclonia.[42] The EEG abnormalities are usually triggered by eye closure, intermittent photic stimulation, and hyperventilation.[42] Fixation-off sensitivity may coexist.[42]

Generalized tonic-clonic seizures

Muscle and movement artifacts mask the EEG during GTCS unless muscle relaxants are used to paralyze the subject. Generalized polyspike-wave bursts usually mark the ictal onset. Generalized amplitude attenuation follows, with or without low voltage, generalized, 20–40 Hz fast activity superimposing for a few seconds. The onset of the tonic phase coincides with the voltage attenuation. Then, generalized rhythmic alpha activity (10–12 Hz) evolves with increasing amplitude and

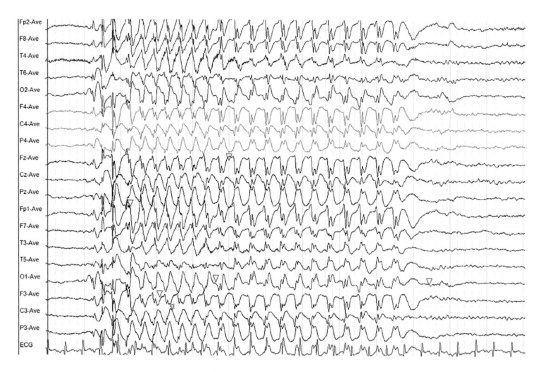

Figure 10.7   EEG of a myoclonic absence seizure. Note the paroxysm of spike-wave discharges is similar to a typical absence seizure as illustrated in Figure 10.4. (Timebase of this EEG = 20 sec/page.)

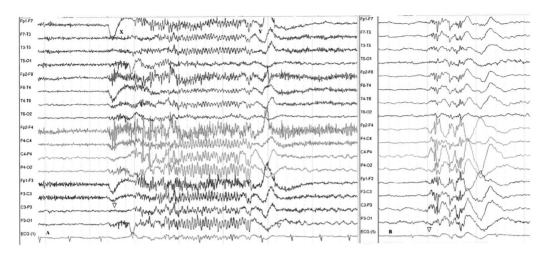

Figure 10.8 **EEG of an absence seizure with eyelid myoclonia in Jeavons syndrome.** (a) The absence seizure was triggered by eye closure at X. Note the paroxysm of generalized, fast polyspike activity (X to Y). This seizure was semiologically characterized by eyelid myoclonus, hyperextension of the neck, and unresponsiveness. (b) Interictal generalized polyspike-wave discharges during sleep recorded from the same patient.

decreasing frequency accompanied by the ongoing tonic phase. When the decreasing frequency reaches 4 Hz, repetitive polyspike-wave complexes emerge accompanied by myoclonic and clonic jerking semiologically. With the progression of the seizure, periodic bursts of polyspike-wave discharges appear with background suppression in between. Generalized EEG suppression is seen for a variable period with the termination of clonic jerking. The gradual recovery is marked by the restoration of the background rhythm from irregular generalized delta slowing proceeding to theta, and finally alpha rhythm (Figure 10.9a–d).[38]

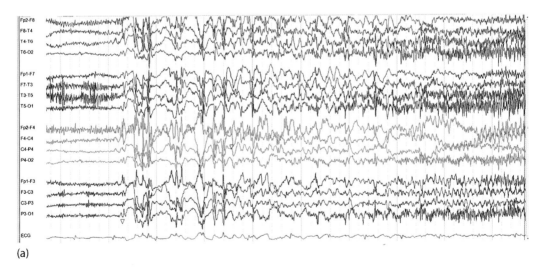

(a)

Figure 10.9 **EEG of a generalized tonic-clinic seizure.** (a) Ictal onset is characterized by bursts of generalized polyspike and wave discharges followed by 12–13 Hz generalized rhythmic alpha activity, indicating the beginning of the tonic phase of the seizure. (b) Evolving ictal rhythm with increasing amplitude and decreasing frequency in the tonic phase. Muscle artifact is beginning to mask the EEG rhythm. (c) The clonic phase of the seizure is characterized by bursts of polyspike and wave discharges with overlapping muscle artifacts. (d) Seizure offset is characterized by bursts of polyspike-wave discharges with overlapping muscle artifacts and background suppression in between. Postictal generalized EEG suppression is also evident. *(Continued)*

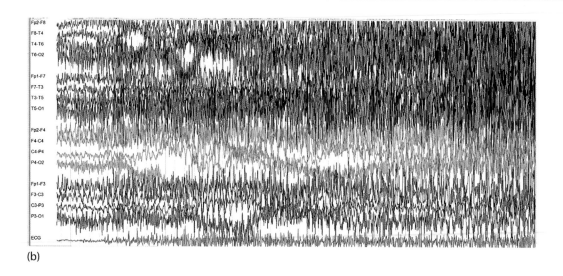

(b)

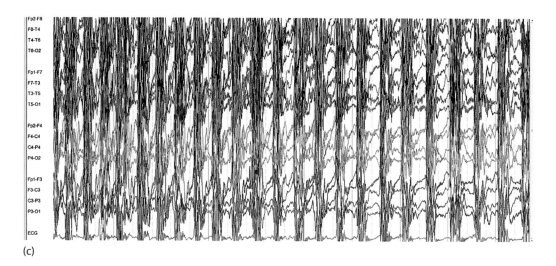

(c)

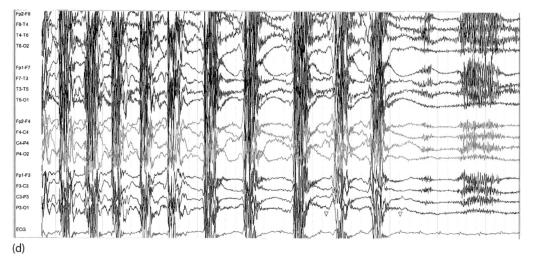

(d)

Figure 10.9   *(Continued)*

ATYPICAL EEG ABNORMALITIES

The typical EEG abnormalities in GGE are generalized, symmetrical, and bisynchronous epileptiform discharges. However, atypical EEG abnormalities such as focal discharges, lateralized discharges, asymmetries, and irregular discharges have been reported in the literature.[43-47] In absence seizures, the initial discharge has been found to be non-generalized in 50%.[36]

A study based on 24-hour ambulatory EEGs has quantified the atypical epileptiform EEG abnormalities in GGE.[48] This study identified six atypical EEG abnormalities: (1) amplitude asymmetry, (2) focal onset of paroxysms, (3) focal offset of paroxysms, (4) focal epileptiform discharges, (5) abnormal morphology, and (6) generalized paroxysmal fast rhythm (Figures 10.10–10.14).

It was found that 66% of GGE patients had at least one type of atypical abnormality in the 24-hour EEG recording. Patients diagnosed with JAE and JME had those abnormalities most frequently, followed by epilepsy with generalized tonic-clonic seizures alone (GTCSA) and CAE. The most frequent atypical abnormality in the cohort was atypical morphology in 93.4% of patients. Other atypical EEG abnormalities were amplitude asymmetry (28%), focal discharges (21.5%), focal onset (13.1%), focal offset (8.2%), and generalized paroxysmal fast rhythm (1.9%).[48] It is of practical relevance to note that atypical abnormalities may result in misdiagnosis and delayed diagnosis.[47]

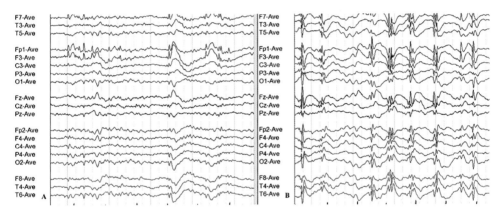

Figure 10.10 Atypical epileptiform discharges: Amplitude asymmetry. (a) Note asymmetric epileptiform discharges with higher amplitude in the left frontal region. Synchronous epileptiform discharges of low amplitude are evident on the right on careful inspection. (b) More symmetric generalized epileptiform discharges recorded from the same patient.

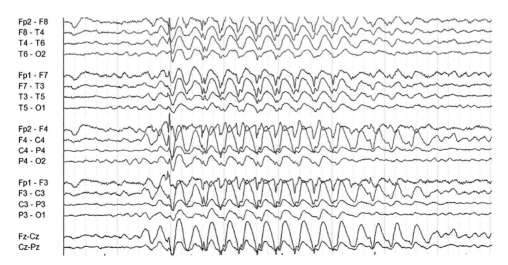

Figure 10.11 Atypical epileptiform discharges: Focal onset and offset of paroxysms. A generalized spike-wave paroxysm in juvenile absence epilepsy. Note the focal onset and offset in the left frontal region.

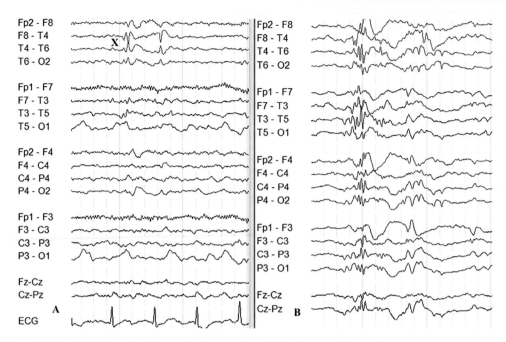

Figure 10.12   Atypical epileptiform discharges: Focal discharges. (a) Note focal discharges at the right temporal region (X). (b) Generalized epileptiform discharges recorded from the same patient.

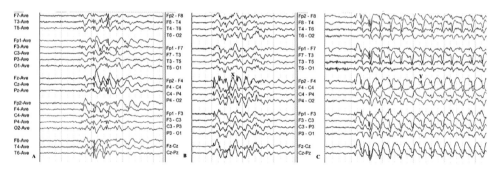

Figure 10.13   Atypical epileptiform discharges: Abnormal morphology. (a) Waves without spikes. Note that at the end of spike-wave paroxysms there are waves without preceding spikes. (b) Spikes overriding the waves. Note the spikes on top of the wave at X. (c) Spikes overriding the waves. Note the spikes on the descending limb of the preceding wave (Y).

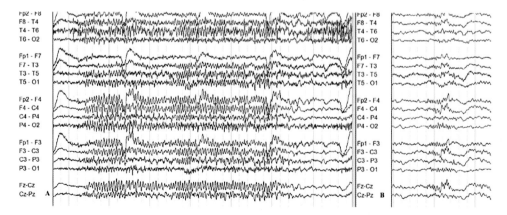

Figure 10.14   Atypical epileptiform discharges: Generalized paroxysmal fast rhythm. (a) A run of generalized fast activity in wakefulness. (b) Similar changes during sleep.

PROVOKING FACTORS AFFECTING THE EEG

Arousals, sleep, sleep deprivation, and circadian rhythmicity

There are circadian variations in seizures and epileptiform discharges in GGE. Generalized spike-wave activity is seen more often in non-rapid eye movement (NREM) sleep, but rare in rapid eye movement (REM) sleep.[49] In GGE, sleep deprivation significantly increases the density of spike-wave discharges in both sleep and wakefulness.[50] In JME, routine EEGs (without sleep deprivation) done in the morning are more often abnormal than those done in the afternoon.[51] In JME, sleep-EEG always shows epileptiform discharges.[52]

Epileptiform discharges in GGE appear to be closely related to the sleep-wake cycle. A retrospective study based on 24-hour ambulatory EEGs found that 4.6% of patients had epileptiform discharges correlating with awakening. All patients who had epileptiform discharges on awakening were diagnosed with GGE. The epileptiform discharges were detected between 20 and 50 minutes following awakening in JME.[53]

The interaction between circadian rhythmicity and the sleep-wake cycle in the generation of epileptiform discharges in GGE has been evaluated in a study.[54] Epileptiform discharges are significantly shorter in duration and more frequent during the NREM sleep compared with wakefulness. When quantified, 67% of epileptiform discharges are detected in NREM sleep, whereas 33% occur in wakefulness. The distribution of epileptiform discharges demonstrates two peaks (11 p.m. to 7 a.m. and 12 noon to 4 p.m.) and two troughs (6 p.m. to 8 p.m. and 9 a.m. to 11 a.m.).[54] These findings highlight the variability in the diagnostic yield in relation to the time of day and sleep-wake cycle. The best time for the optimal yield of EEG abnormalities is from 11 p.m. to 7 a.m. Similarly, capturing natural sleep during the EEG recording significantly increases the diagnostic yield.[54] Hence, 24-hour ambulatory EEG is a very useful diagnostic tool in GGE.

Hyperventilation

Hyperventilation is routinely used as an activation method in EEG. Hyperventilation-induced EEG abnormalities seem to depend on the severity of hypocapnia and the reduction in cerebral blood flow.[55]

Hyperventilation often induces ictal and interictal abnormalities in children diagnosed with absence seizures.[56] Hyperventilation triggered absence seizures in 67% of patients in a pediatric cohort (mean age 9.3 years) diagnosed with JAE and CAE.[55] In untreated children, hyperventilation induced absence seizures more often in CAE and JAE (87% each) in comparison to JME (33%).[7] In contrast, in another study involving a predominantly adult cohort, during hyperventilation, no one with generalized epilepsy had seizures and only 12.2% had an increase in interictal epileptiform discharges.[57] Hyperventilation-induced generalized spike-wave paroxysms were found in only 12.3% of adult patients with GGE on treatment.[13] These studies suggest that during hyperventilation, absence seizures are more likely to occur in the younger age group with untreated CAE and JAE.

Photic stimulation

Intermittent photic stimulation is a routine induction technique during EEG recordings. The photoparoxysmal response is more often seen in generalized epilepsy than in focal epilepsy. It is under the influence of several variables including age, sex, antiepileptic drug (AED) therapy, level of arousal, sleep deprivation, and the stimulation technique.[4]

Reflex triggers

Reflex seizures on exposure to specific stimuli are sometimes encountered in GGE. The use of such stimuli as activating procedures during the EEG recording in selected patients is an option to improve the yield of EEG abnormalities.

Reflex seizures involving visual stimulation have been reported in several epilepsy syndromes including GGE, symptomatic generalized epilepsy, and occipital epilepsy.[58] Flickering lights, patterns, video games, and television are among the common visual triggers. Both photosensitivity and pattern sensitivity are implicated in television- and video-game-induced seizures. Around 90% of patients with electrographic pattern sensitivity also demonstrate photoparoxysmal response.[59] 3-D television and movies do not pose a higher risk of reflex seizures than 2-D television and movies.[60]

Non-verbal cognitive stimuli, such as thinking and praxis, may induce reflex seizures in GGE. In a study involving reflex epilepsy triggered by spatial tasks, card or board games, and calculation, 96% experienced GTCS often preceded by myoclonic jerks, whereas 68% demonstrated generalized epileptiform discharges on EEG.[61] Another study involving 480 patients found that neuropsychological tasks provoked epileptiform discharges in 38 patients and 36 of those patients were diagnosed with GGE.[62] Mental arithmetic and decision-making may trigger "noogenic" (thinking-associated) seizures among susceptible individuals. Cognitive activity in conjunction with planned motor tasks usually with hands is implicated in praxis-induced seizures.[63] Praxis-induced reflex seizures are particularly common in juvenile myoclonic epilepsy.[45,62] Reading, talking and writing are examples of verbal cognitive stimuli that may trigger reflex seizures. Both generalized and focal epilepsies have been reported under this category.[63]

EEG DIFFERENCES AMONG SYNDROMES

Interictal EEG abnormalities in electroclinical syndromes of GGE

Several electroclinical syndromes such as CAE, JAE, JME, and GTCSA have been described in GGE. In this chapter, we will focus on the four main syndromes: CAE, JAE, JME, and GTCSA. It should be noted that apart from the electroclinical syndrome, epileptiform abnormalities in GGE are under the influence of many variables including sex, age, the state of alertness, activation procedures, techniques of EEG recording, and AED therapy.[4]

Interictal EEG in childhood absence epilepsy

CAE is typically seen in children and the EEG signature is "generalized, bisynchronous, and symmetrical 3 Hz spike-wave discharges emerging from a normal background."[2] Fragments of generalized spike-wave discharges are seen in >90% of cases, predominantly in drowsiness and sleep.[7] Interictal polyspikes usually occur in drowsiness and sleep.[7] Polyspike-wave discharges were detected in 26% of patients in a different series.[64] Among untreated children with CAE, only 21% demonstrate photoparoxysmal response, whereas hyperventilation-induced absence seizures are seen in 87%.[7]

OIRDA is seen in 20–30% of CAE subjects,[8,36] and 40% of those have a notched appearance.[36]

Interictal EEG in juvenile absence epilepsy

The onset of JAE is in the teenage years (12–17 years). Absence seizures are less frequent, but myoclonus is more common in JAE compared with CAE. In comparison to CAE, GTCS more frequently precede the onset absence seizures in JAE.[2] Fragmented discharges and polyspikes are seen in all patients, mostly in drowsiness and sleep.[7]

Interictal EEG in juvenile myoclonic epilepsy

Patients with JME typically experience their first seizure at puberty (12–18 years). The typical semiologic feature is myoclonic seizures, predominantly involving arms. GTCS occur more frequently than absences.[2] Sleep deprivation and alcohol are potent seizure triggers. Seizures, particularly myoclonus, frequently occur after awakening from sleep.[19]

The classic EEG abnormalities in JME are generalized polyspikes and polyspike-wave discharges.[19,38] The interictal EEG is characterized by 3–6 Hz spike and polyspike-wave discharges in an irregular mix.[28] Focal EEG abnormalities are common.[45] PPR is seen in the majority.[7] Both eye-closure sensitivity and FOS have been reported in JME.[45]

Interictal EEG in epilepsy with generalized tonic-clonic seizures alone

This condition is characterized by GTCS occurring on awakening or at random times. The median age of onset is (18 years) significantly older than JME and JAE.[65] The interictal EEG demonstrates generalized polyspikes, polyspike-waves, and spike-wave discharges, similar to other GGE syndromes. The mean spike-wave frequency is 3.6 Hz. The density of epileptiform discharges is significantly lower than CAE, JAE, and JME.[66]

CHARACTERISTICS OF ABSENCE SEIZURES IN GGE SYNDROMES

Frequency of GSW discharges

In all GGE syndromes, the initial frequency of GSW activity is faster. In the next phase, the discharges become more regular and slower in frequency by 0.4 to 0.6 Hz. The frequency decreases again in the terminal phase of CAE and JAE.[20] The highest median frequency of GSW during the first second of an absence seizure is in JME (3.5 Hz). It is marginally slower in JAE (3.25 Hz) and CAE (3 Hz).[7] In JME, the generalized spike-wave activity often tends to be faster (>3.5 Hz).[19,38,67] A more recent study based on 24-hour EEGs found median GSW frequencies of 3.3 (CAE), 3.1 (JAE), 3.8 (JME), and 3.5 (GTCSA). But the differences were not statistically significant.[66]

Epileptiform discharge morphology and duration

CAE and JAE demonstrate similar morphologies of GSW discharges. Multiple spikes preceding or overlapping slow waves give rise to an appearance of compressed "W"s in absence seizures of JME.[20] The polyspike-wave activity is seen more often in JME and JAE than in CAE.[7] CAE and JAE have longer EEG seizure durations than JME.[20,68] The longest EEG absence seizure is seen in JAE, whereas the shortest is in GTCSA.[66]

Organization of discharges

Absence seizures typically demonstrate well-organized regular and rhythmic ictal EEG pattern. In disorganized discharges, regular rhythmic activity is interrupted by, (a) brief (<1 sec) and transient interruptions in ictal rhythm, or (b) waveforms of different frequency and/or morphology (Figure 10.15).[7]

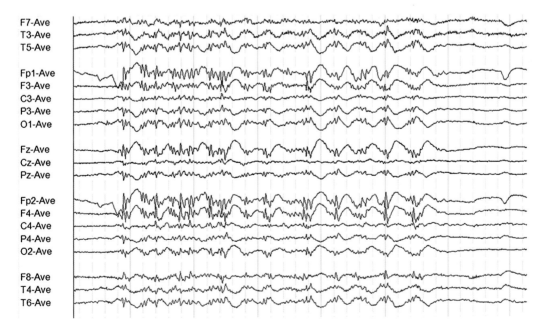

Figure 10.15   A disorganized (irregular) paroxysm of generalized epileptiform discharges in juvenile myoclonic epilepsy. Note this paroxysm has a mix of polyspikes and polyspike-wave discharges with varying frequency and morphology.

Table 10.1 Differences in electroencephalographic features among syndromes

	Reference	CAE	JAE	JME	GTCSA
GSWD frequency (Hz)	66	3.3	3.2	3.9	3.6
Irregular and disorganized paroxysms	7	Least common	8 times more likely than CAE	110 times more likely than CAE	NA
Percentage of GSWD fragments containing polyspikes	7	A: 0, D: 13%, S: 40%	A: 0, D: 12%, S: 24%	A: 50%, D: 50%, S: 50%	NA
Photoparoxysmal response	7	21%	25%	83%	NA
Absence seizures during hyperventilation	7	87%	87%	33%	NA
Mean duration of paroxysms (sec)	66	2.8	4.6	3.2	2.5
Total spike density	66	+	+++	+++	+
Density of generalized paroxysms	66	+	+++	+	+
Density of polyspikes and polyspike-wave discharges	66	+	+++	++	+
Density of pure GSWD	66	++	++	+	+

Abbreviations: CAE: Childhood absence epilepsy; GSWD: Generalized spike-wave discharges; GTCSA: Generalized tonic-clonic seizures alone; JAE: Juvenile absence epilepsy; JME: Juvenile myoclonic epilepsy; NA: Not available; A: Awake; D: Drowsy; S: Sleep; Density: duration of epileptiform discharges (in seconds) per an hour of EEG recording; +++; highest value; +; lowest value; +++; middle value; Pure GSWD: fragments and paroxysms containing only spike-wave discharges (without any polyspikes or polyspike-wave discharges).

Sources: Sadleir LG, et al. EEG features of absence seizures in idiopathic generalized epilepsy: Impact of syndrome, age, and state. Epilepsia 2009; 50(6):1572–1578. Seneviratne U, et al. Can EEG differentiate among syndromes in genetic generalized epilepsy? J Clin Neurophysiol 2017; 34(3):213–221.

Disorganized ictal discharges are 110 times more likely to occur in JME than CAE and eight times more likely in JAE than CAE.[7] It is also influenced by provoking techniques, the state of arousal, and age.[7] Irregular and disorganized paroxysms are also seen in GTCSA, though less frequently.[66]

Table 10.1 summarizes key EEG differences among the four main GGE syndromes.

UNDERPINNING NETWORK MECHANISMS OF GENERALIZED SPIKE-WAVE COMPLEX

Currently, epilepsy is considered a disorder of network pathways. This concept is reflected in the current International League against Epilepsy terminology defining generalized seizures as those involving both cortical and subcortical bilateral networks.[1] Hence, in GGE, the seizure activity originates at a certain point within the epileptic network and then rapidly engages bilaterally distributed network pathways.[1]

Many animal and human experiments highlight the importance of the frontal lobe and thalamus in the formation and propagation of generalized spike-wave complexes. In the rat model, absence seizures originate from the somatosensory cortex rapidly spreading to the thalamus.[69] In their pioneering work, Bancaud and Talairach recorded generalized spike-wave discharges with mesial frontal cortex stimulation.[70] More recently, novel EEG techniques have provided intriguing insights into the underpinning epileptic network pathways in GGE.

Dense array EEG and source localization

A study based on dense array EEG in absence seizures has demonstrated spike-wave discharge onset in the dorsolateral frontal and orbital frontal regions followed by rapid and stereotypic propagation.[71]

Electrical source analysis of dense array EEG data has revealed fronto-temporal networks involving the slow wave and spike propagation through ventromedial frontal networks during absence seizures.[72]

Magnetoencephalography (MEG)/EEG

A combined MEG/EEG study has described a prefrontal-insular-thalamic network in absence epilepsy.[73] In JAE, the spike-wave discharge onset is in focal cortical regions with subsequent involvement of the default mode network as demonstrated by synchronous MEG/EEG data.[74]

Simultaneous EEG and functional MRI (EEG-fMRI) studies

EEG-fMRI is a non-invasive technique to measure regional brain activation during epileptiform discharges using blood oxygenation level-dependent contrast.[75] A recent critical review has elicited three key features among EEG-fMRI findings in GGE: (a) activation of the thalamus, (b) activation of cortical regions, particularly frontal, and (c) deactivation of default mode areas.[47]

Combined transcranial magnetic stimulation and EEG studies

Combined transcranial magnetic stimulation (TMS) and EEG is an emerging non-invasive technique with the potential to study the functional connectivity of the brain.[76] A protocol to study GGE patients with TMS-EEG has been recently described.[77] However, changes in network connectivity have mostly been studied with TMS-EEG in focal epilepsy,[78] while evaluation in GGE remains in its infancy.[79]

Graph theory and EEG

Graph theory is a mathematical concept to study brain connectivity. It describes networks in terms of interrelationship between nodes (brain regions) and edges (connections).[80] Graph theory is increasingly being used as a tool to analyze epileptic networks. One study has reported increased local connectivity in the frontal regions with spike-wave discharges in juvenile myoclonic epilepsy.[81] Another study based on graph theory using EEG data found similarities in network topology between patients with GGE and their unaffected relatives.[82]

Conclusions should be drawn with care from these studies due to various limitations. There is wide variability in the methodology among studies. In particular, EEG-fMRI studies vary in terms of study paradigms, and methods of data acquisition as well as analysis. Additionally, most studies are based on generalized spike-wave activity. In GGE, there are other EEG abnormalities, and underpinning network mechanisms may be different in those. Despite such limitations, there is growing support for the hypothesis that spike-wave discharges originate from a cortical focus with rapid spread to the thalamus followed by entrainment of the cortico-thalamo-cortical loop resulting in the classic generalized spike-wave activity observed in GGE.[83]

DIAGNOSTIC TOOLS

Routine outpatient EEG, sleep-deprived outpatient EEG, short-term outpatient video-EEG, inpatient video-EEG, and 24-hour ambulatory EEG are common tools used to diagnose and classify epilepsy in routine clinical practice. The yield is influenced by several variables such as age, AED therapy, the pretest probability of epilepsy, provoking techniques used, the length of the recording, and the state of arousal.[4]

The yield of interictal epileptiform discharges in the routine outpatient EEG is around 28%.[84] After the first seizure, the average yield is 29% according to a systematic review.[85] Serial EEGs appear to increase the diagnostic yield.[86] One study based on outpatient short-term video-EEG found the yield to be 17.2%.[87] However, in this study, 22% of patients had the test with the clinical diagnosis of psychogenic non-epileptic seizures, reducing the yield of epileptiform discharges. Inpatient video-EEG monitoring has a higher yield (epileptic seizures 43.5%; interictal epileptiform discharges 43%),[88] but is an expensive test with limited availability.

Sleep EEG can be considered the most effective diagnostic tool as 67% of generalized epileptiform discharges occur in NREM sleep.[54] Sleep deprivation appears to increase this yield further. Following sleep deprivation, generalized spike-wave discharge densities increase in both sleep and wakefulness with the highest densities recorded in NREM sleep stages 1 and 2.[50] Though results in the literature are variable, sleep deprivation appears to increase the yield of epileptiform discharges (focal and generalized) by about 30% beyond the effect of sleep.[89]

The use of multiple provoking techniques increases the diagnostic yield of EEG. A study reported a video-EEG protocol incorporating several provoking methods such as sleep deprivation, neuropsychological activation (language and praxis), hyperventilation, eye closure, intermittent photic stimulation, sleep, and arousal.[90] The video-EEG was recorded for 4–6 hours. Interictal epileptiform discharges were detected in 85.8% of patients, whereas 54.9% had seizures during the recording.[90] The high yield might have been influenced by the fact that all patients in the cohort had an established diagnosis of GGE. Yet, this study demonstrates the importance of combining multiple provoking techniques to enhance the diagnostic yield.

Recent research indicates 24-hour ambulatory EEG to be a very useful test to diagnose and classify GGE.[54] Its diagnostic sensitivity is 2.23 times higher than routine EEG.[91] Ambulatory EEG recordings are very effective for several reasons. First, two-thirds of epileptiform discharges appear on sleep EEG recording, and ambulatory EEG is the most practical method to capture natural sleep and increase the diagnostic yield.[54] Second, epileptiform discharges in GGE demonstrates a time-of-day dependence with two peaks (11 p.m. to 7 a.m. and 12 noon to 4 p.m.) and two troughs (6 p.m. to 8 p.m. and 9 a.m. to 11 a.m.).[54] Routine outpatient EEG is likely to miss the most significant first peak (11 p.m. to 7 a.m.) while the 24-hour ambulatory will capture both peaks. Third, it is four times cheaper than inpatient video-EEG.[92] Finally, home-based ambulatory EEG is more convenient and acceptable to patients than hospital-based inpatient monitoring.[93]

DIAGNOSTIC PITFALLS

Misdiagnosis of people without epilepsy as generalized epilepsy

Paroxysmal disorders ranging from syncope to psychogenic non-epileptic seizures can be misdiagnosed as epilepsy. The rate of misdiagnosis is as high as 20–30% in general practice and outpatient clinics.[94,95] Misdiagnosis is likely to happen when an individual presenting with a non-epileptic disorder undergoes an EEG test yielding epileptiform abnormalities. It has been shown that 0.5% of healthy adults in the general population have epileptiform abnormalities in the EEG.[25] Among healthy school children, the prevalence of generalized spike-wave activity in the EEG is 0.9%.[96] Epileptiform discharges are more frequently (37%) detected among the offspring of patients with epilepsy. Six percent of healthy first-degree relatives of JME probands demonstrate typical generalized epileptiform discharges.[97,98] Hence, one must not forget the importance of clinical correlation of EEG abnormalities in establishing the diagnosis of epilepsy.

Misdiagnosis of generalized epilepsy as focal epilepsy

Atypical features, including focal epileptiform discharges, can potentially result in delayed diagnosis and misdiagnosis of GGE. The rate of misdiagnosis can be as high as 91% and the mean delay to the diagnosis ranges from 6 to 15 years in studies.[47] As a result, many patients may receive inappropriate AEDs such as carbamazepine, leading to paradoxical worsening of some seizures.[47]

Misdiagnosis of focal epilepsy as generalized epilepsy

Secondary bilateral synchrony

Tukel and Jasper coined the term "secondary bilateral synchrony" while reporting a series of patients with parasagittal lesions in whom the EEGs demonstrated bilaterally synchronous bursts of spike-wave complexes.[99] Along with Penfield, they postulated that "a cortical focus can fire into subcortical structures and set off a projected secondary bilateral synchrony."[99] Subsequently, a stereo-EEG study reported that stimulation of the mesial frontal region induced paroxysms of bilaterally synchronous and symmetrical spike-wave discharges.[70]

Blume and Pillay proposed three diagnostic criteria for secondary bilateral synchrony: (1) ≥2 seconds of lead-in time, (2) focal triggering spikes having a different morphology from the bisynchronous discharges, and (3) both triggering spikes and focal spikes from the same region have similar morphology.[100] This is a rare phenomenon occurring in 0.5% of patients undergoing EEGs and is most frequently seen in association with frontal lobe foci (Figure 10.16a, b & c).[100]

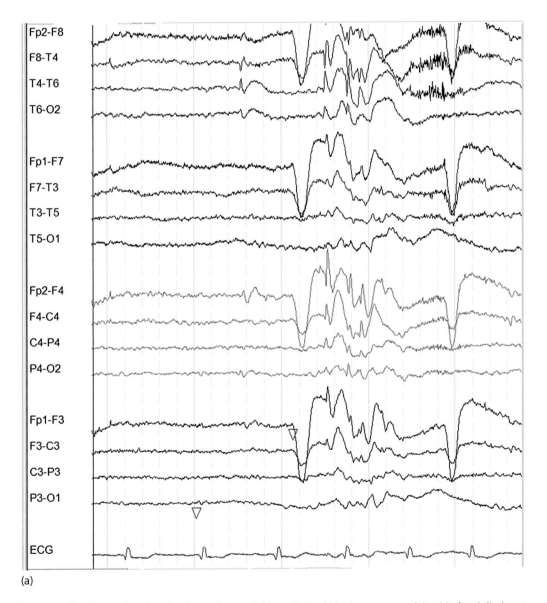

(a)

Figure 10.16   Secondary bilateral synchrony. (a) Longitudinal bipolar montage. A lead-in focal discharge with negative phase reversal is seen at T4 followed by a burst of generalized spike-wave and polyspike-wave discharges. (b) The same EEG segment is displayed on the common average reference montage here. Careful observation reveals amplitude asymmetry of the generalized discharges. (c) An interictal epileptiform discharge captured during the same EEG recording showing a focal epileptiform discharge with amplitude maximum at T4 and similar morphology to the lead-in discharge shown in (a) and (b). *(Continued)*

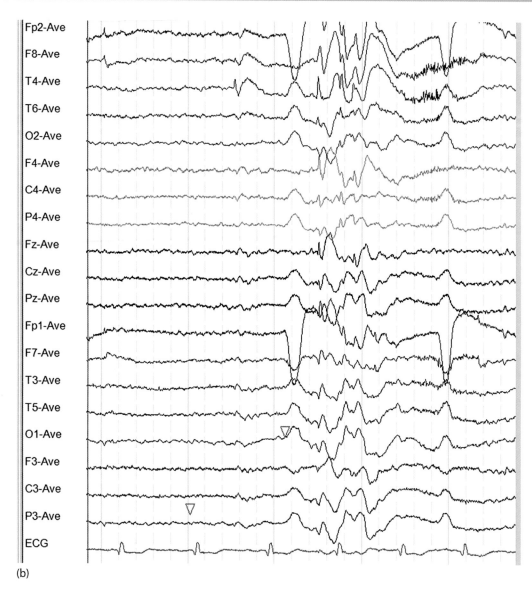

(b)

Figure 10.16 *(Continued)*

Frontal lobe epilepsy: The conundrum of "pseudo bilateral synchrony"

In frontal lobe epilepsy, the interictal epileptiform abnormalities range from focal to bilateral synchronous discharges. In a surgical series of frontal lobe epilepsy, 9% had bifrontal independent interictal epileptiform discharges, whereas bilaterally synchronous discharges were recorded from 37% of patients.[101] Epileptiform discharges recorded on the scalp EEG represent the summated activity of volume conduction and cortico-cortical propagation. Cortico-cortical propagation gives rise to asynchronous discharges with a time lag. However, small time lags may not be appreciated by visual inspection and can be interpreted as synchronous discharges.[102,103] Hence, it is conceivable that frontal foci, particularly located in the midline, can generate bi-frontal epileptiform discharges with "pseudo bilateral synchrony" that can be mistaken for truly bisynchronous discharges of GGE. Computer-aided analysis,[104] or specific re-montaging (reference-subtraction montage)[103] can be used to detect the time lag between the electrodes and demonstrate that bilateral discharges are not truly synchronous but generated from a single focus. Expanding the timebase of digital EEG is also a useful manipulation to detect time differences between seemingly synchronous discharges on two separate channels (Figures 10.17 and 10.18).[105]

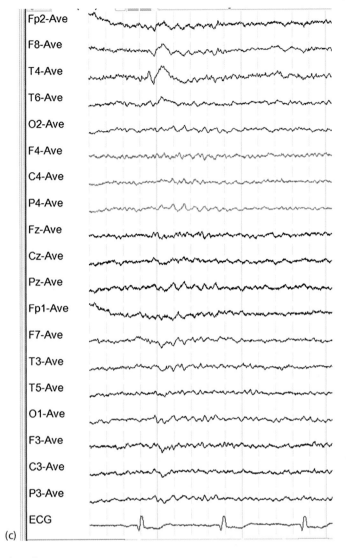

(c)

Figure 10.16 *(Continued)*

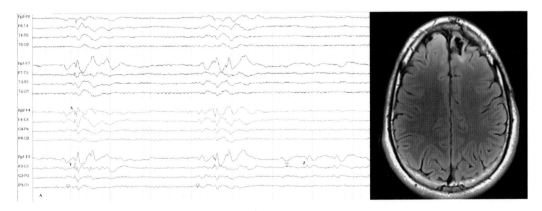

Figure 10.17 Pseudo bilateral synchrony in frontal lobe epilepsy. This patient presented with seizures following the surgery for a left frontal brain abscess in the past. (a) In this longitudinal bipolar montage, bifrontal polyspike-wave discharges (X, Y) appear synchronous. However, focal sharp-wave discharges are evident involving the F3 electrode at Z. (b) The MRI demonstrating left frontal encephalomalacia.

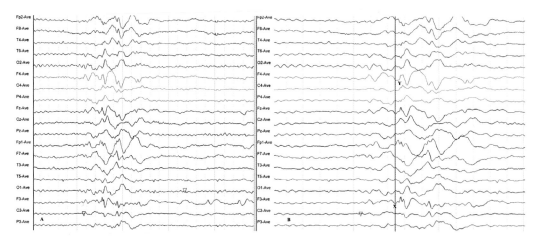

Figure 10.18   Pseudo bilateral synchrony in frontal lobe epilepsy. (a) This average referential montage demonstrates the same activity seen in Figure 10.17. The discharges appear bifrontal. Note focal discharges involving F3 and C3. (Timebase of the EEG = 10 seconds/page) (b) When the timebase is expanded to 5 seconds/page, it becomes clear that the epileptiform discharge emerges first on the left at Fp1 and F3 (X), followed by activity on the right (Y), confirming pseudo bilateral synchrony.

Misdiagnosis of normal variants as generalized epileptiform discharges

The 6 Hz spike-wave (phantom spike-wave) pattern consists of bursts of generalized symmetric spike-wave discharges with a very low amplitude spike component.[106] The bursts are typically very brief but can last up to 4 seconds on rare occasions.[106] The amplitude maxima can be anterior or posterior.[107] This variant, particularly the type with posterior maximum, usually emerges from drowsiness and disappears during deep sleep. Though the typical frequency is 6 Hz, it can range from 4 to 7.5 Hz.[107] The spike component is <25 microvolts in the majority and >75 microvolts in 5%.[107] This is a benign variant of no clinical significance.

The 14 and 6 Hz positive burst pattern (14 and 6 Hz positive spikes or ctenoids) is a benign variant most often seen in early teens, which then becomes infrequent with advancing age. These spikes are surface-positive in polarity, occurring in bursts of <1 second, with unilateral or bilateral distribution and posterior dominance during drowsiness and light sleep.[106] This can be mistaken for polyspikes, but careful analysis of the polarity, frequency, and distribution should help clarify the diagnosis.

Small sharp spikes (benign sporadic sleep spikes) are seen in adults during drowsiness and light sleep. It disappears in deep sleep. The sharp waves are usually diphasic with low amplitude (<50 microvolts) and brief duration (<50 milliseconds) without an after-going slow-wave. The spikes occur in the form of isolated transients with a unilateral or bilateral widespread field most prominent in the temporal regions.[106]

CONCLUSIONS

As highlighted in this chapter, there are several typical EEG features of GGE. The occurrence of atypical features, focal changes in particular, should be borne in mind to avoid misdiagnosis. The use of provoking stimuli such as sleep deprivation, intermittent photic stimulation, hyperventilation, FOS, and reflex triggers during EEG recording can help increase the diagnostic yield. Some EEG features help differentiation among electroclinical syndromes. However, it should be emphasized that such differences are also influenced by several confounding variables including sex, age, state of alertness, activation methods, technical factors, and AED therapy.

This chapter is based on a previous publication: Seneviratne U, Cook MJ, D'Souza WJ. Electroencephalography in the diagnosis of genetic generalized epilepsy syndromes. Front Neurol 2017;8:499.

References

1. Berg, AT, Berkovic, SF, Brodie, MJ, Buchhalter, J, Cross, JH, van Emde Boas, W, et al. Revised terminology and concepts for organization of seizures and epilepsies: Report of the ILAE Commission on Classification and Terminology, 2005–2009. Epilepsia 2010;51:676–685.

2. ILAE. Proposal for revised classification of epilepsies and epileptic syndromes. Commission on Classification and Terminology of the International League Against Epilepsy. Epilepsia 1989;30:389–399.

3. Scheffer, IE, Berkovic, S, Capovilla, G, Connolly, MB, French, J, Guilhoto, L, et al. ILAE classification of the epilepsies: Position paper of the ILAE Commission for Classification and Terminology. Epilepsia 2017;58:512–521.

4. Seneviratne, U, Cook, M, D'Souza, W. The electroencephalogram of idiopathic generalized epilepsy. Epilepsia 2012;53:234–248.

5. Chatrian, GE, Bergamini, L, Dondey, M, Klass, DW, Lennox-Buchthal, M, Petersen, I. A glossary of terms most commonly used by clinical electroencephalographers. Electroencephalogr Clin Neurophysiol 1974;37:538–548.

6. Blumenfeld, H. Consciousness and epilepsy: Why are patients with absence seizures absent? Prog Brain Res 2005;150:271–286.

7. Sadleir, LG, Scheffer, IE, Smith, S, Carstensen, B, Farrell, K, Connolly, MB. EEG features of absence seizures in idiopathic generalized epilepsy: Impact of syndrome, age, and state. Epilepsia 2009; 50:1572–1578.

8. Dlugos, D, Shinnar, S, Cnaan, A, Hu, F, Moshe, S, Mizrahi, E, et al. Pretreatment EEG in childhood absence epilepsy: Associations with attention and treatment outcome. Neurology 2013;81:150–156.

9. Gibbs, FA, Davis, H, Lennox, WG. The electro-encephalogram in epilepsy and in conditions of impaired consciousness. Arch Neurol Psychiatry 1935;34:1133–1148.

10. Gibbs, FA, Gibbs, EL, Lennox, WG. Epilepsy: A paroxysmal cerebral dysrhythmia. Brain 1937;60:377–388.

11. Weir, B The morphology of the spike-wave complex. Electroencephalogr Clin Neurophysiol 1965;19: 284–290.

12. Blume, WT, Lemieux, JF. Morphology of spikes in spike-and-wave complexes. Electroencephalogr Clin Neurophysiol 1988;69:508–515.

13. Seneviratne, U, Cook, M, D'Souza, W. Consistent topography and amplitude symmetry are more typical than morphology of epileptiform discharges in genetic generalized epilepsy. Clin Neurophysiol 2016;127:1138–1146.

14. Lemieux, JF, Blume, WT. Topographical evolution of spike-wave complexes. Brain Res 1986;373: 275–287.

15. Clemens, B, Bessenyei, M, Piros, P, Toth, M, Seress, L, Kondakor, I. Characteristic distribution of interictal brain electrical activity in idiopathic generalized epilepsy. Epilepsia 2007;48:941–949.

16. Rodin, E, Ancheta, O. Cerebral electrical fields during petit mal absences. Electroencephalogr Clin Neurophysiol 1987;66:457–466.

17. Holmes, MD, Quiring, J, Tucker, DM. Evidence that juvenile myoclonic epilepsy is a disorder of fronto-temporal corticothalamic networks. Neuroimage 2010;49:80–93.

18. da Silva Braga, AM, Fujisao, EK, Betting, LE. Analysis of generalized interictal discharges using quantitative EEG. Epilepsy Res 2014;108:1740–1747.

19. Delgado-Escueta, AV, Enrile-Bacsal, F. Juvenile myoclonic epilepsy of Janz. Neurology 1984;34:285–294.

20. Panayiotopoulos, CP, Obeid, T, Waheed, G. Differentiation of typical absence seizures in epileptic syndromes. A video EEG study of 224 seizures in 20 patients. Brain 1989;112(Pt 4):1039–1056.

21. Markand, ON. Lennox-Gastaut syndrome (childhood epileptic encephalopathy). J Clin Neurophysiol 2003;20:426–441.

22. Markand, ON. Pearls, perils, and pitfalls in the use of the electroencephalogram. Semin Neurol 2003;23:7–46.

23. Kasteleijn-Nolst Trenite, DG, Guerrini, R, Binnie, CD, Genton, P. Visual sensitivity and epilepsy: A proposed terminology and classification for clinical and EEG phenomenology. Epilepsia 2001;42:692–701.

24. Puglia, JF, Brenner, RP, Soso, MJ. Relationship between prolonged and self-limited photoparoxysmal responses and seizure incidence: Study and review. J Clin Neurophysiol 1992;9:137–144.

25. Gregory, RP, Oates, T, Merry, RT. Electroencephalogram epileptiform abnormalities in candidates for aircrew training. Electroencephalogr Clin Neurophysiol 1993;86:75–77.

26. Kooi, KA, Thomas, MH, Mortenson, FN. Photoconvulsive and photomyoclonic responses in adults. An appraisal of their clinical significance. Neurology 1960;10:1051–1058.

27. Brandt, H, Brandt, S, Vollmond, K. EEG response to photic stimulation in 120 normal children. Epilepsia 1961;2:313–317.

28. Panayiotopoulos, CP. Syndromes of idiopathic generalized epilepsies not recognized by the International League Against Epilepsy. Epilepsia 2005;46(Suppl 9):57–66.

29. Panayiotopoulos, CP. Fixation-off, scotosensitive, and other visual-related epilepsies. Adv Neurol 1998;75:139–157.

30. Koutroumanidis, M, Tsatsou, K, Sanders, S, Michael, M, Tan, SV, Agathonikou, A, et al. Fixation-off sensitivity in epilepsies other than the idiopathic epilepsies of childhood with occipital paroxysms: A 12-year clinical-video EEG study. Epileptic Disord 2009;11:20–36.

31. Agathonikou, A, Koutroumanidis, M, Panayiotopoulos, CP. Fixation-off (scoto) sensitivity combined with photosensitivity. Epilepsia 1998;39:552–555.

32. Niedermeyer, E. Sleep electroencephalograms in petit mal. Arch Neurol 1965;12:625–630.

33. Niedermeyer, E. Primary (idiopathic) generalized epilepsy and underlying mechanisms. Clin Electroencephalogr 1996;27:1–21.

34. Seneviratne, U, Cook, M, D'Souza, W. Epileptiform K-complexes and sleep spindles: An underreported phenomenon in genetic generalized epilepsy. J Clin Neurophysiol 2016;33:156–161.

35. Riviello, JJ Jr., Foley, CM. The epileptiform significance of intermittent rhythmic delta activity in childhood. J Child Neurol 1992;7:156–160.

36. Sadleir, LG, Farrell, K, Smith, S, Connolly, MB, Scheffer, IE. Electroclinical features of absence seizures in childhood absence epilepsy. Neurology 2006;67:413–418.

37. Janz, D. Epilepsy with impulsive petit mal (juvenile myoclonic epilepsy). Acta Neurol Scand 1985; 72:449–459.

38. Hrachovy, RA, Frost, JD Jr. The EEG in selected generalized seizures. J Clin Neurophysiol 2006; 23: 312–332.

39. Drury, I, Henry, TR. Ictal patterns in generalized epilepsy. J Clin Neurophysiol 1993;10:268–280.

40. ILAE. Proposal for revised clinical and electroencephalographic classification of epileptic seizures. From the Commission on Classification and Terminology of the International League Against Epilepsy. Epilepsia 1981;22:489–501.

41. Bureau, M, Tassinari, CA. Epilepsy with myoclonic absences. Brain Dev 2005;27:178–184.

42. Giannakodimos, S, Panayiotopoulos, CP. Eyelid myoclonia with absences in adults: A clinical and video-EEG study. Epilepsia 1996;37:36–44.

43. Lombroso, CT. Consistent EEG focalities detected in subjects with primary generalized epilepsies monitored for two decades. Epilepsia 1997;38:797–812.

44. Matur, Z, Baykan, B, Bebek, N, Gurses, C, Altindag, E, Gokyigit, A. The evaluation of interictal focal EEG findings in adult patients with absence seizures. Seizure 2009;18:352–358.

45. Panayiotopoulos, CP, Obeid, T, Tahan, AR. Juvenile myoclonic epilepsy: A 5-year prospective study. Epilepsia 1994;35:285–296.

46. Panayiotopoulos, CP, Tahan, R, Obeid, T. Juvenile myoclonic epilepsy: Factors of error involved in the diagnosis and treatment. Epilepsia 1991;32:672–676.

47. Seneviratne, U, Cook, M, D'Souza, W. Focal abnormalities in idiopathic generalized epilepsy: A critical review of the literature. Epilepsia 2014;55:1157–1169.

48. Seneviratne, U, Hepworth, G, Cook, M, D'Souza, W. Atypical EEG abnormalities in genetic generalized epilepsies. Clin Neurophysiol 2016;127:214–220.

49. Martins da Silva, A, Aarts, JH, Binnie, CD, Laxminarayan, R, Lopes da Silva, FH, Meijer, JW, et al. The circadian distribution of interictal epileptiform EEG activity. Electroencephalogr Clin Neurophysiol 1984;58:1–13.

50. Halasz, P, Filakovszky, J, Vargha, A, Bagdy, G. Effect of sleep deprivation on spike-wave discharges in idiopathic generalised epilepsy: A 4 × 24 h continuous long term EEG monitoring study. Epilepsy Res 2002;51:123–132.

51. Labate, A, Ambrosio, R, Gambardella, A, Sturniolo, M, Pucci, F, Quattrone, A. Usefulness of a morning routine EEG recording in patients with juvenile myoclonic epilepsy. Epilepsy Res 2007;77:17–21.

52. Dhanuka, AK, Jain, BK, Daljit, S, Maheshwari, D. Juvenile myoclonic epilepsy: A clinical and sleep EEG study. Seizure 2001;10:374–378.

53. Fittipaldi, F, Curra, A, Fusco, L, Ruggieri, S, Manfredi, M. EEG discharges on awakening: A marker of idiopathic generalized epilepsy. Neurology 2001;56:123–126.

54. Seneviratne, U, Boston, RC, Cook, M, D'Souza, W. Temporal patterns of epileptiform discharges in genetic generalized epilepsies. Epilepsy Behav 2016;64:18–25.

55. Wirrell, EC, Camfield, PR, Gordon, KE, Camfield, CS, Dooley, JM, Hanna, BD. Will a critical level of hyperventilation-induced hypocapnia always induce an absence seizure? Epilepsia 1996;37:459–462.

56. Dalby, MA. Epilepsy and 3 per second spike and wave rhythms. A clinical, electroencephalographic and prognostic analysis of 346 patients. Acta Neurol Scand 1969:Suppl 40:43+.

57. Holmes, MD, Dewaraja, AS, Vanhatalo, S. Does hyperventilation elicit epileptic seizures? Epilepsia 2004;45:618–620.

58. Zifkin, BG, Kasteleijn-Nolst Trenite, D. Reflex epilepsy and reflex seizures of the visual system: A clinical review. Epileptic Disord 2000;2:129–136.

59. Radhakrishnan, K, St Louis, EK, Johnson, JA, McClelland, RL, Westmoreland, BF, Klass, DW. Pattern-sensitive epilepsy: Electroclinical characteristics, natural history, and delineation of the epileptic syndrome. Epilepsia 2005;46:48–58.

60. Prasad, M, Arora, M, Abu-Arafeh, I, Harding, G. 3D movies and risk of seizures in patients with photosensitive epilepsy. Seizure 2012;21:49–50.

61. Goossens, LA, Andermann, F, Andermann, E, Remillard, GM. Reflex seizures induced by calculation, card or board games, and spatial tasks: A review of 25 patients and delineation of the epileptic syndrome. Neurology 1990;40:1171–1176.

62. Matsuoka, H, Takahashi, T, Sasaki, M, Matsumoto, K, Yoshida, S, Numachi, Y, et al. Neuropsychological EEG activation in patients with epilepsy. Brain 2000;123 (Pt 2):318–330.

63. Ferlazzo, E, Zifkin, BG, Andermann, E, Andermann, F. Cortical triggers in generalized reflex seizures and epilepsies. Brain 2005;128:700–710.

64. Vierck, E, Cauley, R, Kugler, SL, Mandelbaum, DE, Pal, DK, Durner, M. Polyspike and waves do not predict generalized tonic-clonic seizures in childhood absence epilepsy. J Child Neurol 2010;25: 475–481.

65. Vorderwulbecke, BJ, Kowski, AB, Kirschbaum, A, Merkle, H, Senf, P, Janz, D, et al. Long-term outcome in adolescent-onset generalized genetic epilepsies. Epilepsia 2017.

66. Seneviratne, U, Hepworth, G, Cook, M, D'Souza, W. Can EEG differentiate among syndromes in genetic generalized epilepsy? J Clin Neurophysiol 2017;34:213–221.

67. Montalenti, E, Imperiale, D, Rovera, A, Bergamasco, B, Benna, P. Clinical features, EEG findings and diagnostic pitfalls in juvenile myoclonic epilepsy: A series of 63 patients. J Neurol Sci 2001;184: 65–70.

68. Sadleir, LG, Scheffer, IE, Smith, S, Carstensen, B, Carlin, J, Connolly, MB, et al. Factors influencing clinical features of absence seizures. Epilepsia 2008;49:2100–2107.

69. Meeren, HK, Pijn, JP, Van Luijtelaar, EL, Coenen, AM, Lopes da Silva, FH. Cortical focus drives widespread corticothalamic networks during spontaneous absence seizures in rats. J Neurosci 2002; 22:1480–1495.

70. Bancaud, J, Talairach, J, Morel, P, Bresson, M, Bonis, A, Geier, S, et al. "Generalized" epileptic seizures elicited by electrical stimulation of the frontal lobe in man. Electroencephalogr Clin Neurophysiol 1974;37:275–282.

71. Holmes, MD, Brown, M, Tucker, DM. Are "generalized" seizures truly generalized? Evidence of localized mesial frontal and frontopolar discharges in absence. Epilepsia 2004;45:1568–1579.

72. Tucker, DM, Brown, M, Luu, P, Holmes, MD. Discharges in ventromedial frontal cortex during absence spells. Epilepsy Behav 2007;11:546–557.

73. Stefan, H, Paulini-Ruf, A, Hopfengartner, R, Rampp, S. Network characteristics of idiopathic generalized epilepsies in combined MEG/EEG. Epilepsy Res 2009;85:187–198.

74. Sakurai, K, Takeda, Y, Tanaka, N, Kurita, T, Shiraishi, H, Takeuchi, F, et al. Generalized spike-wave discharges involve a default mode network in patients with juvenile absence epilepsy: A MEG study. Epilepsy Res 2010;89:176–184.

75. Hamandi, K, Salek-Haddadi, A, Laufs, H, Liston, A, Friston, K, Fish, DR, et al. EEG-fMRI of idiopathic and secondarily generalized epilepsies. Neuroimage 2006;31:1700–1710.

76. Ilmoniemi, RJ, Kicic, D. Methodology for combined TMS and EEG. Brain Topogr 2010;22:233–248.

77. Kimiskidis, VK, Tsimpiris, A, Ryvlin, P, Kalviainen, R, Koutroumanidis, M, Valentin, A, et al. TMS combined with EEG in genetic generalized epilepsy: A phase II diagnostic accuracy study. Clin Neurophysiol 2017;128:367–381.

78. Kugiumtzis, D, Kimiskidis, VK. Direct causal networks for the study of transcranial magnetic stimulation effects on focal epileptiform discharges. Int J Neural Syst 2015;25:1550006.

79. Fadini, T, Nitsche, M, Paulus, W. Tracing origin and propagation areas of epileptic activity by combining TMS and EEG source analysis in generalized epilepsy. Epilepsia 2009;50:186–187.

80. Bernhardt, BC, Bonilha, L, Gross, DW. Network analysis for a network disorder: The emerging role of graph theory in the study of epilepsy. Epilepsy Behav 2015;50:162–170.

81. Lee, C, Im, CH, Koo, YS, Lim, JA, Kim, TJ, Byun, JI, et al. Altered network characteristics of spike-wave discharges in juvenile myoclonic epilepsy. Clin EEG Neurosci 2017;48:111–117.

82. Chowdhury, FA, Woldman, W, FitzGerald, TH, Elwes, RD, Nashef, L, Terry, JR, et al. Revealing a brain network endophenotype in families with idiopathic generalised epilepsy. PLoS One 2014;9:e110136.

83. Stefan, H, Lopes da Silva, FH. Epileptic neuronal networks: Methods of identification and clinical relevance. Front Neurol 2013;4:8.

84. Angus-Leppan, H. Seizures and adverse events during routine scalp electroencephalography: A clinical and EEG analysis of 1000 records. Clin Neurophysiol 2007;118:22–30.

85. Krumholz, A, Wiebe, S, Gronseth, G, Shinnar, S, Levisohn, P, Ting, T, et al. Practice parameter: Evaluating an apparent unprovoked first seizure in adults (an evidence-based review): Report of the Quality Standards Subcommittee of the American Academy of Neurology and the American Epilepsy Society. Neurology 2007;69:1996–2007.

86. Betting, LE, Mory, SB, Lopes-Cendes, I, Li, LM, Guerreiro, MM, Guerreiro, CA, et al. EEG features in idiopathic generalized epilepsy: Clues to diagnosis. Epilepsia 2006;47:523–528.

87. Seneviratne, U, Rahman, Z, Diamond, A, Brusco, M. The yield and clinical utility of outpatient short-term video-electroencephalographic monitoring: A five-year retrospective study. Epilepsy Behav 2012; 25:303–306.

88. Ghougassian, DF, d'Souza, W, Cook, MJ, O'Brien, TJ. Evaluating the utility of inpatient video-EEG monitoring. Epilepsia 2004;45:928–932.

89. Ellingson, RJ, Wilken, K, Bennett, DR. Efficacy of sleep deprivation as an activation procedure in epilepsy patients. J Clin Neurophysiol 1984;1:83–101.

90. De Marchi, LR, Corso, JT, Zetehaku, AC, Uchida, CGP, Guaranha, MSB, Yacubian, EMT. Efficacy and safety of a video-EEG protocol for genetic generalized epilepsies. Epilepsy Behav 2017;70:187–192.

91. Keezer, MR, Simard-Tremblay, E, Veilleux, M. The diagnostic accuracy of prolonged ambulatory versus routine EEG. Clinl EEG Neurosci 2016;47:157–161.

92. Faulkner, HJ, Arima, H, Mohamed, A. The utility of prolonged outpatient ambulatory EEG. Seizure 2012;21:491–495.

93. Seneviratne, U, Mohamed, A, Cook, M, D'Souza, W. The utility of ambulatory electroencephalography in routine clinical practice: A critical review. Epilepsy Res 2013;105:1–12.

94. Scheepers, B, Clough, P, Pickles, C. The misdiagnosis of epilepsy: Findings of a population study. Seizure 1998;7:403–406.

95. Smith, D, Defalla, BA, Chadwick, DW. The misdiagnosis of epilepsy and the management of refractory epilepsy in a specialist clinic. Q J Med 1999;92:15–23.

96. Okubo, Y, Matsuura, M, Asai, T, Asai, K, Kato, M, Kojima, T, et al. Epileptiform EEG discharges in healthy children: Prevalence, emotional and behavioral correlates, and genetic influences. Epilepsia 1994;35:832–841.

97. Delgado-Escueta, AV, Greenberg, D, Weissbecker, K, Liu, A, Treiman, L, Sparkes, R, et al. Gene Mapping in the idiopathic generalized epilepsies: Juvenile myoclonic epilepsy, childhood absence epilepsy, epilepsy with grand mal seizures, and early childhood myoclonic epilepsy. Epilepsia 1990;31 Suppl 3:S19–29.

98. Jayalakshmi, SS, Mohandas, S, Sailaja, S, Borgohain, R. Clinical and electroencephalographic study of first-degree relatives and probands with juvenile myoclonic epilepsy. Seizure 2006;15:177–183.

99. Tukel, K, Jasper, H. The electroencephalogram in parasagittal lesions. Electroencephalogr Clin Neurophysiol 1952;4:481–494.

100. Blume, WT, Pillay, N. Electrographic and clinical correlates of secondary bilateral synchrony. Epilepsia 1985;26:636–641.

101. Quesney, LF. Preoperative electroencephalographic investigation in frontal lobe epilepsy: Electroencephalographic and electrocorticographic recordings. Can J Neurol Sci 1991;18:559–563.

102. Jayakar, P, Duchowny, M, Resnick, TJ, Alvarez, LA. Localization of seizure foci: Pitfalls and caveats. J Clin Neurophysiol 1991;8:414–431.

103. Jayakar, P, Duchowny, MS, Resnick, TJ, Alvarez, LA. Localization of epileptogenic foci using a simple reference-subtraction montage to document small interchannel time differences. J Clin Neurophysiol 1991;8:212–215.

104. Gotman, J. Measurement of small time differences between EEG channels: Method and application to epileptic seizure propagation. Electroencephalogr Clin Neurophysiol 1983;56:501–514.

105. Seneviratne, U. Rational manipulation of digital EEG: Pearls and pitfalls. J Clin Neurophysiol 2014; 31:507–516.

106. Klass, DW, Westmoreland, BF. Nonpileptogenic epileptiform electroencephalographic activity. Ann Neurol 1985;18:627–635.

107. Hughes, JR. Two forms of the 6/sec spike and wave complex. Electroencephalogr Clin Neurophysiol 1980;48:535–550.

CHAPTER 11

EEG of focal epilepsies

The current International League Against Epilepsy (ILAE) position paper provides a three-tier framework to classify epilepsies.[1] The first tier is based on the classification of seizures into focal, generalized, and unknown types. In keeping with the seizure types, the second tier consists of epilepsy types: generalized, focal, combined generalized and focal, and unknown. In the third tier, epilepsy types are classified into epilepsy syndromes. Running alongside these tiers are the etiologies of epilepsies ranging from structural, genetic, immune, metabolic, and infectious to unknown. Seizure semiology, electroencephalogram (EEG), and neuroimaging play crucial roles in this classification.

Detailed discussions on all focal epilepsy types are beyond the scope of this book. Hence, in this chapter, we will discuss selected focal epilepsy types commonly encountered in clinical practice.

MESIAL TEMPORAL LOBE EPILEPSY

The most common pathology of mesial temporal lobe epilepsy (MTLE) is hippocampal sclerosis (HS), whilst other causes include tumors and gliosis following trauma and infections. Familial cases have also been described. Some patients have dual pathology characterized by HS and another lesion. Patients with HS-associated MTLE often have a history of initial precipitating incidents, such as febrile convulsions, trauma, hypoxia, and cerebral infections during childhood, usually before 5 years of age.[2] Those who are refractory to antiepileptic drug therapy are candidates for epilepsy surgery (anterior temporal lobectomy). Early identification of refractory patients is very important and epilepsy surgery is superior to prolonged drug therapy in those cases.[3]

The typical seizure semiology consists of an aura followed by behavioral arrest, altered awareness, and automatisms in the form of focal unaware (complex partial) seizures. Focal to bilateral tonic-clonic (secondarily generalized) seizures and status epilepticus are rare.[4] Ninety-six percent of patients experience auras and the most frequent are abdominal visceral sensations (nausea, butterflies, rising epigastric sensation) followed by fear, anxiety, *Déjà vu*, gustatory, and olfactory sensations.[4] Oroalimentary (repetitive lip-smacking, chewing, swallowing) and manual (picking, fumbling) automatisms are typical. Autonomic manifestations, such as pupillary dilatation, tachycardia, and piloerection, may also be seen.

The neuroimaging modality of choice is magnetic resonance imaging (MRI) to demonstrate evidence of hippocampal sclerosis. Interictal fluorodeoxyglucose-positron emission tomography (FDG-PET) scans are also useful to demonstrate concordant hypometabolism in the same region. Neuropsychological testing is required in the presurgical workup to elicit memory, intellectual,

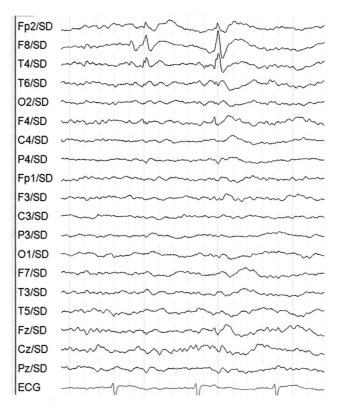

Figure 11.1 Interictal epileptiform discharges in right mesial temporal lobe epilepsy with hippocampal sclerosis.

and language deficits. Typically, episodic memory rather than semantic memory is impaired in MTLE. Verbal memory deficits usually lateralize to the dominant hemisphere, whereas non-verbal memory deficits indicate non-dominant temporal lobe involvement.

The typical interictal EEG hallmark is surface-negative sharp waves or sharp and slow waves with anterior temporal maxima (F7/F8) (Figure 11.1). Other non-specific interictal findings include irregular temporal slowing and temporal intermittent rhythmic delta activity (Figure 11.2).

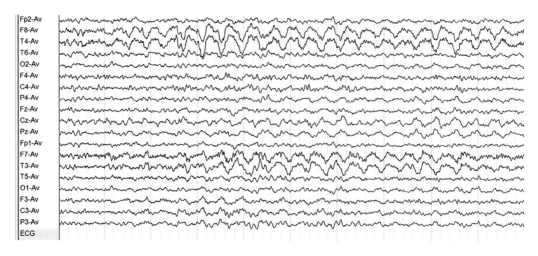

Figure 11.2 Temporal intermittent rhythmic delta activity (bilateral).

During long-term monitoring, independent bilateral anterior temporal discharges are seen in some patients with unilateral HS, which is not considered a contraindication for epilepsy surgery. However, it should be kept in mind that HS can be bilateral.

The interictal epileptiform discharges may attenuate or stop leading up to the seizure. In the ictal EEG, the ictal onset is often marked by focal or lateralized attenuation of the EEG activity. In the typical ictal rhythm, rhythmic theta activity appears over the anterior temporal region, followed by a gradual increase in amplitude and decrease in frequency while spreading to other electrodes (Figure 11.3a–d).[2]

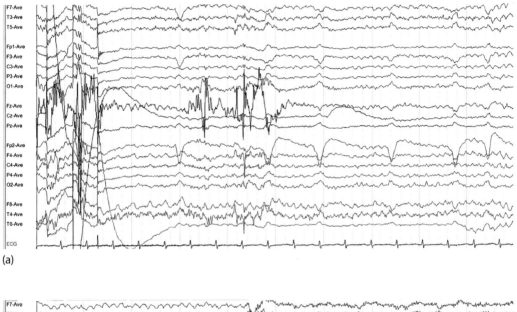

(a)

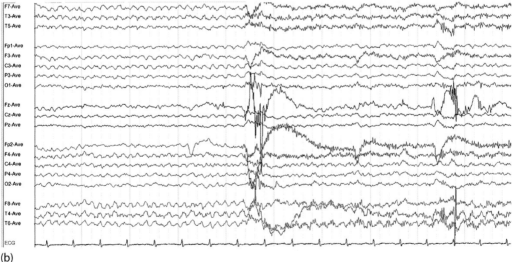

(b)

Figure 11.3 **"Recruiting ictal rhythm" recorded from a patient with right mesial temporal lobe epilepsy with hippocampal sclerosis.** (a) Ictal onset with rhythmic theta activity over F8T4 electrodes. (b) Evolving rhythm: Rhythmic theta slows down toward the end of the epoch. (c) Further evolution: Rhythmic delta with gradually increasing amplitude over F8T4T6. (d) Further evolution of the ictal rhythm with propagation to the left hemisphere. *(Continued)*

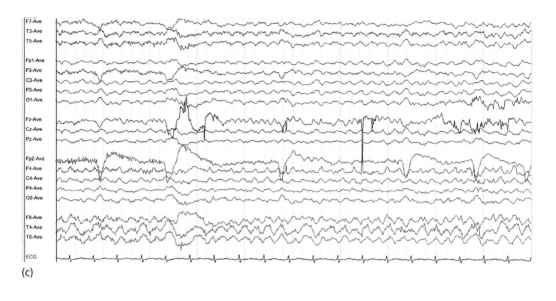

(c)

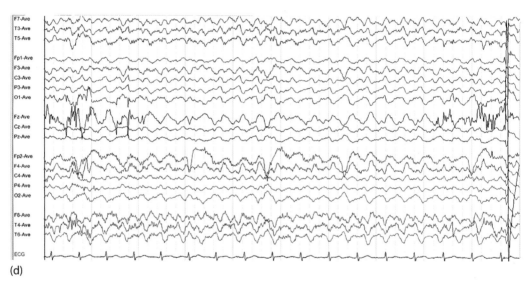

(d)

Figure 11.3   *(Continued)*

Although the typical seizure-onset pattern is rhythmic theta activity, ictal onset with rhythmic alpha and delta has been described (Figure 11.4a–c).[5] Ictal discharges remain localized to the anterior and mesial regions in the vast majority whilst hemispherical and non-localizing discharges are seen occasionally.[5] Propagation to the contralateral hemisphere occurs in <50% after a median time of 10 seconds. The clinical seizure onset precedes the ictal surface EEG onset in 53%.[5] Several other ictal rhythms such as repetitive spiking, widespread theta, and "start-stop-start phenomenon" have been described. Post-ictal slowing has a high lateralizing value.

NEOCORTICAL (LATERAL) TEMPORAL LOBE EPILEPSY

Seizures in neocortical temporal lobe epilepsy (NTLE) originate from the lateral neocortex of the temporal lobe. Underlying pathologies include malformations of cortical development, neoplasms, gliosis, and vascular malformations. About 60% of patients experience auras such as auditory,

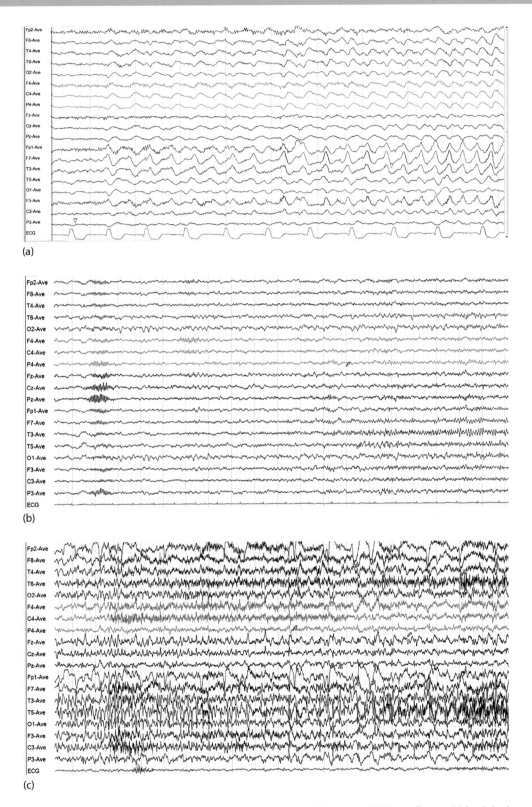

Figure 11.4   Ictal onset with non-theta frequencies in mesial temporal lobe epilepsy. (a) Ictal rhythm recorded from a patient with left mesial temporal lobe epilepsy with hippocampal sclerosis. Note the ictal onset with rhythmic delta activity over F7T3 electrodes. (b) Ictal onset with rhythmic alpha frequency in left mesial temporal lobe epilepsy with hippocampal sclerosis. (c) Note evolving ictal rhythm and timebase is compressed to 30 sec/page.

vertiginous, psychic phenomena, and abdominal visceral sensations. Gustatory and olfactory auras are rare. Loss of contact (motionless unresponsiveness) is often the first and earliest sign within 10 seconds of seizure onset.[6] Secondarily, generalized tonic-clonic seizures are more common in NTLE than in MTLE. Seizure duration is shorter in NTLE.

Interictal epileptiform discharges do not significantly differ from MTLE, though lateralized slow waves and epileptiform discharges tend to be more frequent in NTLE.[7] The discharges are usually maximal at anterior and mid-temporal electrodes (Figure 11.5a & b).

The early ictal rhythm was reported to be slower (2–5 Hz) and more widespread (lateralized versus anterior temporal) compared with MTLE.[8] However, contradicting results have been reported in more-recent studies. One such study found rhythmic theta ictal rhythm in 49% of seizures (Figure 11.6) compared with 22% of rhythmic delta and 15% of faster (beta) rhythms in NTLE seizures.[9]

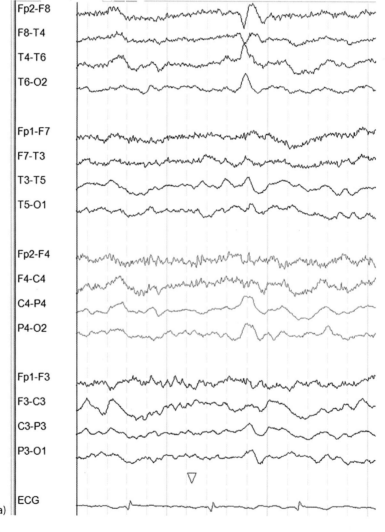

(a)

Figure 11.5 Interictal epileptiform discharges in lateral temporal lobe epilepsy. (a) Negative phase reversal of a sharp wave at the T4 electrode on the longitudinal bipolar montage. (b) Same epoch displayed on the average referential montage confirms the amplitude maximum over T4. An MRI brain scan of the patient shows focal cortical dysplasia of the right middle temporal gyrus. *(Continued)*

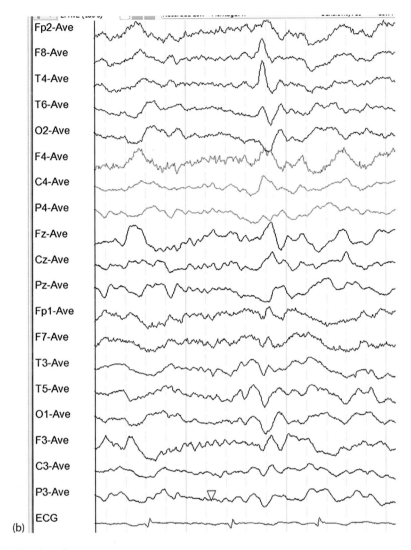

Figure 11.5   (Continued)

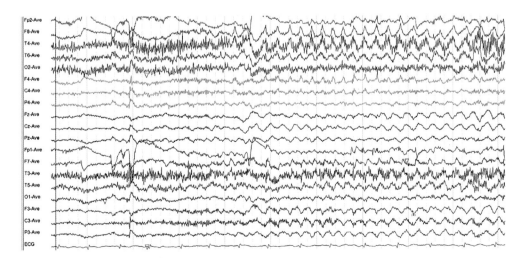

Figure 11.6   Ictal rhythm of a seizure recorded from the patient discussed in Figure 11.5. Note ictal onset with rhythmic theta activity over the T4 electrode.

FRONTAL LOBE EPILEPSY

The frontal lobe is a complex region, rich in connections, that gives rise to a wide spectrum of semiologies. Tumors, malformations of cortical development, vascular malformations including cavernomas, and post-traumatic gliosis are common etiologies. Genetic frontal-lobe epilepsies are rare and autosomal dominant nocturnal frontal-lobe epilepsy is a classic example.

Anatomically, it is divided into several regions such as pre-central (lateral and medial), pre-motor (lateral and medial), pre-frontal (dorsolateral, ventrolateral, frontopolar), and orbitofrontal. Amongst diverse semiological presentations, some common features are evident in seizures of frontal-lobe origin. Seizures are usually brief with sudden onset and offset with a tendency for clustering and fast secondary generalization. Motor manifestations are very frequent whilst postictal confusion is minimal. Complex gestural automatisms and behaviors including hyperkinetic movements are very characteristic. Bilateral asymmetric tonic seizures are the hallmark of seizures originating from the supplementary motor area of the mesial frontal lobe. Akinetic seizures are witnessed when the onset is in the negative motor area. A more detailed discussion of semiology is beyond the scope of this book.

Up to 40% do not show interictal epileptiform discharges.[10] The field of epileptiform discharges tends to be widespread and bilateral, sometimes mimicking generalized epilepsy. Focal discharges are more commonly encountered with lateral frontal foci.[10] Paradoxical lateralization may occur with midline frontal foci as explained previously. The epileptiform discharges appear in the form of spikes, spike-wave activity, sharp waves, sharp and slow waves, and paroxysmal fast activity. Rhythmic midline theta activity during wakefulness can be a useful marker.

The ictal EEG is often masked by muscle artifacts as the motor activity often occurs very early in frontal lobe seizures. With seizures of lateral frontal onset, the typical ictal rhythms are characterized by repetitive spiking, rhythmic fast activity, and rhythmic delta activity. Bilateral low voltage fast activity, often preceded by a high-amplitude sharp transient, is seen in the fronto-central leads during mesial frontal seizures (Figure 11.7 a & b).

PARIETAL LOBE EPILEPSY

The typical aura of parietal lobe epilepsy is characterized by contralateral somatosensory disturbances in the form of numbness, tingling, thermal sensation, or pain. Rarely, the somatosensory

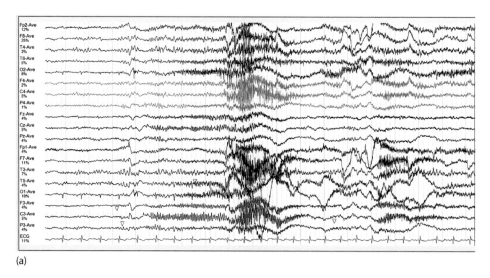

(a)

Figure 11.7 Ictal rhythm in mesial frontal-lobe epilepsy in a patient with asymmetric tonic seizures arising from the left supplementary motor area (timebase compressed to 20 sec/page). (a) Note rhythmic fast activity involving the F3C3 electrodes in a subtle seizure captured in sleep. (b) A typical asymmetric tonic seizure. The ictal onset is characterized by a direct current shift (slow wave) followed by fast activity in the left fronto-central region. Further evolution of the ictal rhythm is mostly masked by the muscle artifacts. *(Continued)*

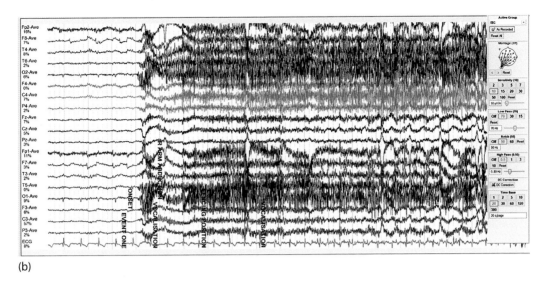

(b)

Figure 11.7   *(Continued)*

aura can be ipsilateral or bilateral.[11] Other auras include body image disturbance, moving sensation, vertiginous sensation, and visual auras, particularly when the precuneus region of the posterior medial parietal cortex is involved. Other ictal manifestations are usually due to the propagation of the seizure activity and include motor, versive, hyperkinetic, and automotor seizures.[11]

The interictal epileptiform discharges may be seen in the fronto-parietal, parieto-occipital, temporo-parietal, fronto-centro-parietal, or posterior head regions. Secondary bilateral synchrony is seen in 31%.[12] Localization of the ictal activity is poor and seen in only 10%.[13] False lateralization and localization in parietal-lobe epilepsy is well known and most patients may end up with invasive intracranial EEG monitoring to delineate the seizure onset zone in the surgical workup.

OCCIPITAL LOBE EPILEPSY

The etiologies of occipital epilepsies include malformations of cortical development, neoplasms, trauma, vascular (such as Sturge-Weber syndrome), stroke, metabolic (e.g., mitochondrial disorders, Celiac disease), neurodegenerative (e.g., progressive myoclonic epilepsies), and genetic.[14] Idiopathic generalized epilepsies may have overlapping features with idiopathic occipital epilepsies.

The key semiological feature is visual hallucinations. Three types of visual hallucinations have been described: (1) elementary – flashes of light, spots, blobs, (2) intermediary – geometric shapes (kaleidoscope effect, stars, circles etc.), and (3) complex – objects, humans, and animals.[15] Elementary visual hallucinations arising from the visual cortex are characterized by flashes of light, spots, or blobs. Spinning and rotatory movements are rarely seen. Negative phenomena include amaurosis, hemianopia, and scotomas. Occipital seizures can be misdiagnosed as migraine due to these features. Elementary visual hallucinations can be generated outside the primary visual cortex in lingual and fusiform gyri. Intermediary hallucinations predominantly arise from the right hemisphere in the infra-calcarine occipital cortex anterior to the origin of elementary hallucinations.[15] More complex formed visual hallucinations originate from the occipito-temporal cortex. Kinetopsia (visual illusion of movement) usually localizes to the lateral occipital cortex and the occipito-temporal junction. Other manifestations of occipital seizures include nystagmus, tonic eye deviation, and eyelid fluttering. Anterior and superior seizure propagation gives rise to additional semiologies, such as sensory, motor, and complex partial seizures.

Discrete occipital spikes and paroxysms are the electrographic hallmarks of occipital epilepsy. Occipital photoparoxysmal response and fixation-off sensitivity may be seen in some occipital epilepsies, particularly idiopathic type. The ictal rhythm may manifest as repetitive spiking or evolving fast activity.

There are three idiopathic occipital syndromes particularly important in childhood. Gastaut-type idiopathic occipital epilepsy manifests around 3–15 years of age (mean 8 years) with brief elementary visual hallucinations, tonic eye deviation, and ictal blindness. The EEG demonstrates occipital spikes and fixation off sensitivity. Idiopathic photosensitive occipital epilepsy presents around the same age with reflex seizures triggered by visual stimuli including video games. The EEG shows the occipital photoparoxysmal response. Panayiotopoulos syndrome starts around 3–6 years of age, presenting with autonomic seizures and autonomic status epilepticus.[16]

INSULAR EPILEPSY

The insula is considered the fifth lobe of the brain, lying deep to the Sylvian fissure enclosed by the frontal, parietal, and temporal opercula. It has widespread connections to several key regions of the brain. Anatomically, the insula is divided into two parts, anterior and posterior, separated by the central sulcus of the insula. The anterior insula consists of three short gyri (anterior, middle, and posterior) and an accessory gyrus whilst two long gyri (anterior and posterior) comprise the posterior insula.

The complex semiology of insular seizures reflects its rich somatosensory, motor, viscerosensory, visceromotor, autonomic, and auditory functional representations and connections. Somatosensory auras, usually bilateral, are the most frequent and may be painful. Compared with somatosensory auras from the primary sensory cortex (parietal), insular auras usually involve a larger area and do not follow the typical Jacksonian march. Somatosensory auras usually localize to the posterior insula. Visceral sensory (abdominal sensation, chest tightness, throat constriction, choking), visceral motor (belching, gagging, vomiting), vegetative/psychic (breathlessness, anxiety, fear) auras, and hyperkinetic seizures suggest an anterior insular onset. Additionally, asymmetric tonic seizures, ipsilateral eye blinking, vestibular/auditory auras, and autonomic disturbances are well recognized in insular epilepsy.[17,18]

Due to its deep location, insular epilepsy may not show any interictal epileptiform discharges on the surface EEG. When it does show, the discharges may be recorded from frontal, temporal, and central leads. Anterior insular foci are associated with interictal epileptiform discharges over Fp1/Fp2, F7/F8, C3/C4, T3/T4, and T5/T6 electrodes, whilst posterior insular foci show involvement of T3/T4, T5/T6, and F7/F8 electrode involvement.[19] Ictal EEG may be masked by muscle and movement artifacts. Ictal changes are usually seen over frontal, temporal, and central regions, but can be non-lateralizing. The ictal rhythm may appear in the form of low-voltage fast activity, rhythmic spike-wave, rhythmic alpha, or rhythmic delta waves with lateralized onset or bilateral onset with ipsilateral predominance.

BENIGN CENTROTEMPORAL (ROLANDIC) EPILEPSY OF CHILDHOOD

This childhood epilepsy syndrome is worth discussing under the umbrella of focal epilepsies. The onset is usually between 2 and 13 years of age, and the seizures typically go into remission before or during adolescence.[20] Though the neuropsychiatric profile of the patients is usually reported normal,[20] detailed testing may reveal deficits. Seizures characterized by hemifacial twitching, hemiclonic activity of arms or legs, unilateral perioral numbness, speech arrest, guttural sounds, and hypersalivation typically occur out of sleep or immediately after awakening. Seizures are usually brief and infrequent. Though secondary generalization may occur, status epilepticus is rare. Postictal neurological deficits are observed in 80%.[21]

Interictal EEG

The interictal epileptiform discharges demonstrate certain typical characteristics which help the reader confirm the diagnosis in the correct clinical context.

a. Morphology of sharp and slow wave complex. The sharp and slow wave complex is characterized by a prominent high-amplitude (>200 microvolts) surface-negative sharp wave with a blunt peak, preceded by a low-amplitude (<10 microvolts) positivity, followed by a prominent positivity (with amplitude up to 50% of the negative sharp wave) and a surface-negative slow wave

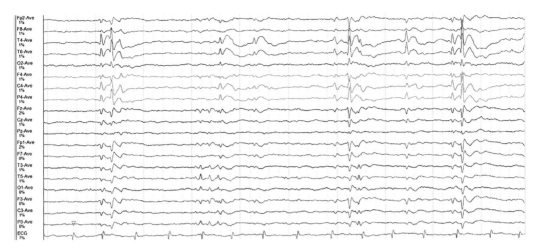

Figure 11.8   Typical interictal epileptiform discharges in benign Rolandic epilepsy.

with an amplitude less than the negative sharp wave (Figure 11.8).[22] The morphology and the topography remain consistent throughout the EEG of a given subject.

b. Topography. The maximum negativity of the sharp wave is seen over the mid-temporal (T3/T4), high-central (C3/C4), low-central (C5/C6), or, occasionally, parietal (P3P4) regions.[21,22] The discharges may be ipsilateral or contralateral to the symptomatogenic zone. Bilateral independent as well as bilateral synchronous epileptiform discharges are not uncommon.

c. Field. It is typical to find a tangential dipole with maximum negativity over the central or centrotemporal regions and maximum positivity over the frontal regions (Figure 11.8). This dipole is thought to represent a source located in the lower part of the Rolandic fissure.

d. Reactivity. Sleep activates the epileptiform discharges in this condition. The amplitude, field of distribution, and frequency of discharges increase as well as become periodic with NREM sleep. On the contrary, contralateral hand movements may attenuate the discharges.[22]

Ictal EEG

Four ictal EEG patterns have been described: (1) Low voltage fast rhythmic spikes increasing in amplitude and decreasing in frequency, (2) spikes and sharp waves increasing in amplitude and frequency, (3) rhythmic theta activity increasing in amplitude and decreasing in frequency, and (4) focal attenuation followed any of the three patterns described above.[23]

It is important to emphasize that typical Rolandic spikes may be seen in perfectly healthy children who may never experience seizures. Centrotemporal spikes can also be seen in some epileptic encephalopathies as well as structural lesions in the Rolandic area. Hence, the significance of this EEG finding should always be interpreted in the clinical context.

References

1. Scheffer, IE, Berkovic, S, Capovilla, G, et al. ILAE classification of the epilepsies: Position paper of the ILAE Commission for Classification and Terminology. Epilepsia 2017;58:512–521.

2. Weiser, HG. Mesial temporal lobe epilepsy with hippocampal sclerosis. Epilepsia 2004;45:695–714.

3. Wiebe, S, Blume, WT, Girvin, JP, Eliasziw, M. A randomized, controlled trial of surgery for temporal-lobe epilepsy. N Engl J Med 2001;345:311–318.

4. French, JA, Williamson, PD, Thadani, VM, et al. Characteristics of medial temporal lobe epilepsy: I. Results of history and physical examination. Ann Neurol 1993;34:774–780.

5. Malter, MP, Bahrenberg, C, Niehusmann, P, Elger, CE, Surges, R. Features of scalp EEG in unilateral mesial temporal lobe epilepsy due to hippocampal sclerosis: Determining factors and predictive value for epilepsy surgery. Clin Neurophysiol 2016;127:1081–1087.

6. Maillard, L, Vignal, JP, Gavaret, M, et al. Semiologic and electrophysiologic correlations in temporal lobe seizure subtypes. Epilepsia 2004;45:1590–1599.

7. O'Brien, TJ, Kilpatrick, C, Murrie, V, Vogrin, S, Morris, K, Cook, MJ. Temporal lobe epilepsy caused by mesial temporal sclerosis and temporal neocortical lesions. A clinical and electroencephalographic study of 46 pathologically proven cases. Brain 1996;119(Pt 6):2133–2141.

8. Foldvary, N, Lee, N, Thwaites, G, et al. Clinical and electrographic manifestations of lesional neocortical temporal lobe epilepsy. Neurology 1997;49:757–763.

9. Lee, SK, Kim, JY, Hong, KS, Nam, HW, Park, SH, Chung, CK. The clinical usefulness of ictal surface EEG in neocortical epilepsy. Epilepsia 2000;41:1450–1455.

10. Kellinghaus, C, Luders, HO. Frontal lobe epilepsy. Epileptic Disord 2004;6:223–239.

11. Kim, DW, Lee, SK, Yun, CH, et al. Parietal lobe epilepsy: The semiology, yield of diagnostic workup, and surgical outcome. Epilepsia 2004;45:641–649.

12. Salanova, V, Andermann, F, Rasmussen, T, Olivier, A, Quesney, LF. Parietal lobe epilepsy. Clinical manifestations and outcome in 82 patients treated surgically between 1929 and 1988. Brain 1995; 118(Pt 3):607–627.

13. Williamson, PD, Boon, PA, Thadani, VM, et al. Parietal lobe epilepsy: Diagnostic considerations and results of surgery. Ann Neurol 1992;31:193–201.

14. Taylor, I, Scheffer, IE, Berkovic, SF. Occipital epilepsies: Identification of specific and newly recognized syndromes. Brain 2003;126:753–769.

15. Jonas, J, Frismand, S, Vignal, JP, et al. Right hemispheric dominance of visual phenomena evoked by intracerebral stimulation of the human visual cortex. Hum Brain Mapp 2014;35:3360–3371.

16. Adcock, JE, Panayiotopoulos, CP. Occipital lobe seizures and epilepsies. J Clin Neurophysiol 2012; 29:397–407.

17. Obaid, S, Zerouali, Y, Nguyen, DK. Insular epilepsy: Semiology and noninvasive investigations. J Clin Neurophysiol 2017;34:315–323.

18. Peltola, ME, Trebuchon, A, Lagarde, S, et al. Anatomoelectroclinical features of SEEG-confirmed pure insular-onset epilepsy. Epilepsy Behav 2020;105:106964.

19. Levy, A, Yen Tran, TP, Boucher, O, Bouthillier, A, Nguyen, DK. Operculo-insular epilepsy: Scalp and intracranial electroencephalographic findings. J Clin Neurophysiol 2017;34:438–447.

20. Beaussart, M. Benign epilepsy of children with Rolandic (centro-temporal) paroxysmal foci. A clinical entity. Study of 221 cases. Epilepsia 1972;13:795–811.

21. Berroya, AM, Bleasel, AF, Stevermuer, TL, Lawson, J, Bye, AME. Spike morphology, location, and frequency in benign epilepsy with centrotemporal spikes. J Child Neurol 2005;20:188–194.

22. Pan, A, Lüders, HO. Epileptiform discharges in benign focal epilepsy of childhood. Epileptic Disord 2000;2(Suppl 1):S29–36.

23. Capovilla, G, Beccaria, F, Bianchi, A, et al. Ictal EEG patterns in epilepsy with centro-temporal spikes. Brain Dev 2011;33:301–309.

CHAPTER 12

EEG of developmental and epileptic encephalopathies

Developmental and epileptic encephalopathies typically present in childhood, but eventually are seen in adult epilepsy clinics as children grow up. Ongoing epileptic activity is considered a contributory factor to cognitive, developmental, and behavioral impairment in these patients. Underlying etiologies vary, ranging from genetic to structural causes. A detailed discussion of the many syndromes in this group is beyond the scope of this book. Two syndromes of infantile-onset (West syndrome and Dravet syndrome) and childhood-onset (Lennox-Gastaut syndrome [LGS] and Landau-Kleffner syndrome) are discussed in this chapter as representative examples.

WEST SYNDROME

Clinical

Typically beginning in infancy, West syndrome is characterized by the triad of epileptic spasms, hypsarrhythmia (on electroencephalogram), and psychomotor retardation. Epileptic spasms can be flexor and/or extensor with unilateral, bilateral symmetric, or bilateral asymmetric distribution.[1] Some go on to develop LGS later in childhood.

Interictal EEG

The interictal EEG hallmark is hypsarrhythmia. It is characterized by high-amplitude (>300 μV), disorganized, slow background admixed with often asynchronous multifocal spike and sharp waves over both hemispheres, most abundant and prominent during NREM sleep (Figure 12.1).

Ictal EEG

The most frequent and earliest change is high-amplitude, frontally dominant, generalized slow wave with or without overriding fast activity. Diffuse-fast activity or electrodecremental response may follow the slow wave (Figure 12.2). Generalized slow wave followed by electrodecrement is the most common pattern, whereas generalized sharp and slow wave followed by electrodecrement is relatively less frequent. The slow wave, fast rhythm, or electrodecremental response can also occur in isolation.[1] The hypsarrhythmia pattern tends to wane between epileptic spasms.

DRAVET SYNDROME

Clinical

Also known as severe myoclonic epilepsy in infancy, Dravet syndrome is a rare epileptic encephalopathy in which seizures begin in infancy usually between 5 and 8 months of age. The SCN1A gene mutation has been identified in 70–80% of cases. The first seizure is typically triggered by

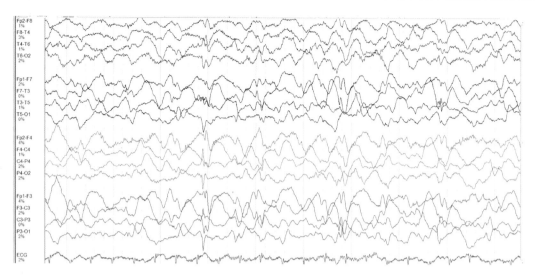

Figure 12.1 Hypsarrhythmia in West syndrome.

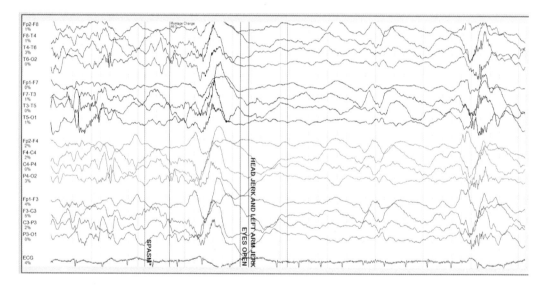

Figure 12.2 Ictal EEG of a spasm characterized by generalized slow wave with overriding fast activity followed by electrodecrement in West syndrome.

vaccination or fever, but is longer than usual febrile convulsions and characterized by unilateral or generalized clonic activity. The development is usually normal until the first seizure and slows down after that. The first seizure is followed by recurrent multiple seizure types including simple focal, complex partial, myoclonic, clonic, generalized tonic-clinic, atypical absence, atonic, tonic (rarely), and status epilepticus often triggered by fever. Phenytoin, carbamazepine, and lamotrigine tend to exacerbate seizures. The long-term prognosis of the condition is poor, and seizures are usually drug-resistant.

Interictal EEG

The background may be normal or slow in the early stages. Rhythmic theta activity, triggered by eye closure, is seen over the central regions and vertex in some cases.[2] Paroxysms of generalized spike wave and fast polyspike wave discharges with fronto-central maxima are seen.

Additionally, there are focal and multifocal spikes and polyspikes.[2] Electrographic photosensitivity, with or without accompanying clinical events, is common. Some patients exhibit pattern sensitivity. Epileptiform abnormalities become more active during NREM sleep.

Ictal EEG

The ictal EEG pattern depends on the seizure type. Myoclonic seizures are accompanied by brief (<10 seconds) generalized spike-wave discharges with fronto-central maxima followed by slow waves. The ictal rhythm of atypical absences consists of irregular, generalized slow spike-wave (SSW) discharges of 2–3.5 Hz.[2] Tonic seizures are uncommon in Dravet syndrome and, when present, the ictal rhythm may manifest as generalized fast activity, electrodecremental response, or a rapid recruiting rhythm.[2]

LENNOX-GASTAUT SYNDROME

Clinical

LGS is a severe form of childhood encephalopathy characterized by the triad of (1) multiple seizure types, (2) generalized slow spike-and-wave (SSW) activity in wakefulness and paroxysmal fast activity in sleep, and (3) cognitive and behavioral impairment. The typical age of onset is 1 to 8 years. Tonic seizures are the most frequent. Other seizure types include atypical absences as well as atonic, myoclonic, generalized tonic-clonic, and focal seizures. Nonconvulsive status epilepticus is common. Seizures are usually drug-resistant and very frequent.

Interictal EEG

a. The EEG background is usually slow to varying degrees. Generalized slowing is seen in up to 90% of patients.[3]

b. The SSW activity, characterized by a sharp wave, a spike, or a polyspike followed by a surface-negative slow wave occurring at 1.5–2 Hz is the electrographic hallmark of LGS (Figure 12.3).[3,4] The SSW complexes occur as isolated discharges or paroxysmal runs. The discharges tend to be generalized and bisynchronous with frontal or frontocentral maxima. The frequency, morphology, and amplitude tend to vary within and between paroxysms. Amplitude asymmetries between the hemispheres are not uncommon. SSW activity is markedly increased during NREM sleep. Photic stimulation and hyperventilation generally have no impact on SSW activity.

c. Focal and multifocal epileptiform discharges are seen in approximately 18% of patients.[3]

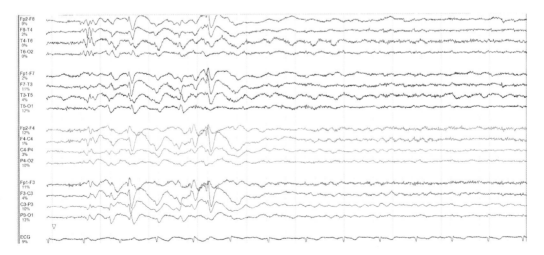

Figure 12.3   Generalized slow spike-wave discharges in Lennox-Gastaut syndrome.

Ictal EEG

a. Tonic seizures: Tonic seizures appear with axial (head and torso), extremities (particularly arms), or whole-body involvement. Generalized paroxysmal fast activity (GPFA) and electrodecremental response are the key ictal rhythms associated with tonic seizures (see Chapter 9 for details). These key rhythms appear in the form of four major ictal rhythms in LGS:[3] (1) Generalized electrodecremental response with no other activity (Figure 12.4), (2) GPFA of 15–25 Hz with progressively increasing amplitude, (3) GPFA of 10–15 Hz without amplitude evolution (Figure 12.5), and (4) electrodecremental response followed by GPFA.

b. Atypical absences: Compared with typical absences of childhood absence epilepsy, the impairment of awareness in atypical absences is partial and progressive. They tend to have a longer duration with a gradual onset and offset.[5] Automatisms are less frequent, whilst decreases or increases in tone occur more often during atypical absences.[5] Furthermore, compared with typical absences, atypical absence seizures are less likely to be triggered by hyperventilation and photic stimulation. The ictal EEG is characterized by generalized, high-amplitude, 1.5–2.5 Hz SSW discharges (Figure 12.6a & b). Compared with the interictal SSW, the ictal rhythm tends to be higher in amplitude, more symmetrical, more regular, better sustained, and longer in duration, though it does not reach the morphology and rhythmicity of a typical absence seizure (Figure 12.6c).[4]

c. Atonic seizures: Epileptic drop attacks in LGS are due to atonic, myoclonic, myoclonic-atonic, or tonic seizures. Pure atonic seizures are rare. The ictal rhythm consists of generalized polyspike-wave discharges of SSW activity followed by generalized slow waves.

d. Myoclonic seizures: The ictal rhythm is characterized by irregular generalized polyspike wave activity.

e. Status epilepticus: Status epilepticus usually consists of atypical absences and tonic seizures manifesting with clouding of consciousness. The ictal rhythm is characterized by generalized and persistent irregular SSW patterns often resembling hypsarrhythmia.

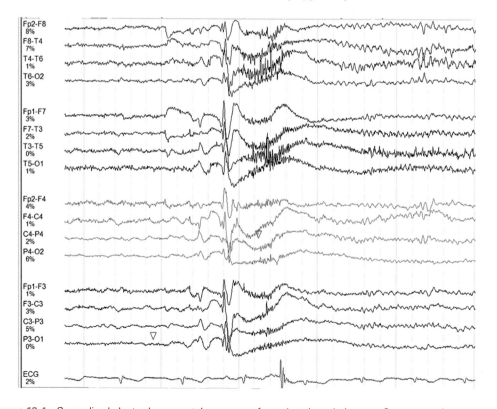

Figure 12.4   Generalized electrodecremental response of a tonic seizure in Lennox-Gastaut syndrome.

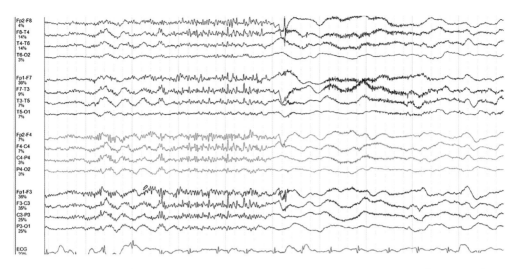

Figure 12.5 Generalized paroxysmal fast activity associated with a tonic seizure in Lennox-Gastaut syndrome.

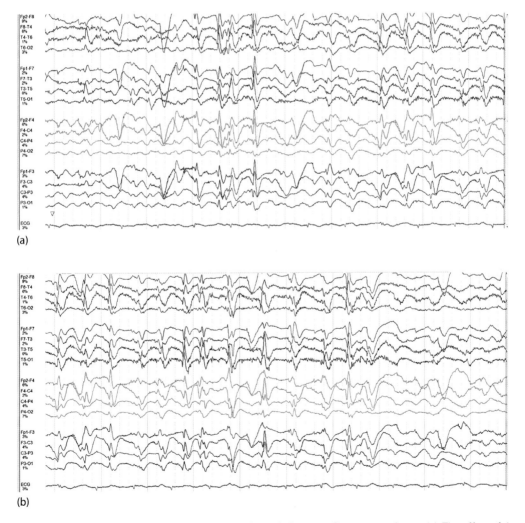

(a)

(b)

Figure 12.6   The onset of an atypical absence seizure in Lennox-Gastaut syndrome (a). The offset of the atypical absence seizure (b). A typical absence seizure in idiopathic generalized epilepsy (c) is shown here for comparison with (a) and (b). *(Continued)*

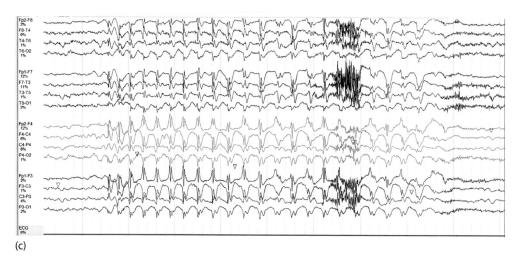

(c)

Figure 12.6   *(Continued)*

LANDAU-KLEFFNER SYNDROME

Clinical

Also known as acquired epileptic aphasia, Landau-Kleffner syndrome is a rare epileptic encephalopathy characterized by acquired aphasia and sleep-activated epileptiform paroxysms accompanied by psychomotor disturbances. The typical age of onset is 3–9 years of age, up to which the development is normal. Auditory verbal agnosia or "word deafness" is usually the first presenting symptom. The language disturbance can progress to total mutism and fluctuations are well known in Landau-Kleffner syndrome. Seizures are experienced by 70% of patients, often going into remission by 15 years of age. The spectrum of seizures includes simple focal (often nocturnal), generalized tonic-clonic, atypical absence, and myoclonic-astatic seizures. Tonic and complex partial seizures are rare.[6] The prognosis is variable with complete language recovery reported in some cases.

EEG

The interictal EEG consists of sharp and slow wave or spike and wave discharges over the temporal and temporoparietal regions. The discharges may be unilateral, multifocal, bilateral independent, or synchronous (Figure 12.7).[7] This activity is significantly activated by NREM sleep,

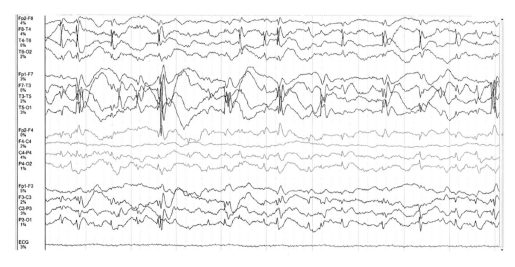

Figure 12.7   Interictal epileptiform discharges in Landau-Kleffner syndrome.

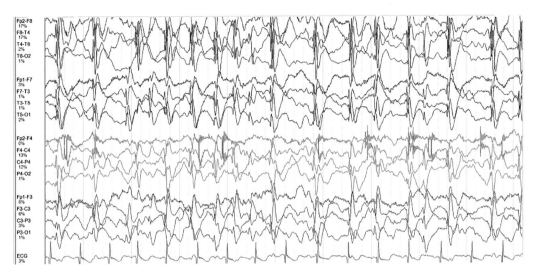

Figure 12.8 Electrical status epilepticus during non-rapid eye movement sleep recorded from the same patient (in Figure 12.7).

particularly at sleep onset. In NREM sleep, some children develop electrical status epilepticus characterized by continuous bilateral 1.5–2.5 Hz SSW activity occupying >85% of the sleep EEG (Figure 12.8).[8]

References

1. Kellaway, P, Hrachovy, RA, Frost, JD Jr, Zion, T. Precise characterization and quantification of infantile spasms. Ann Neurol 1979;6:214–218.

2. Bureau, M, Bernardina, BD. Electroencephalographic characteristics of Dravet syndrome. Epilepsia 2011;52:13–23.

3. Markand, ON. Lennox-Gastaut syndrome (childhood epileptic encephalopathy). J Clin Neurophysiol 2003;20:426–441.

4. Markand, ON. Slow spike-wave activity in EEG and associated clinical features: Often called 'Lennox' or 'Lennox-Gastaut' syndrome. Neurology 1977;27:746–757.

5. Holmes, GL, McKeever, M, Adamson, M. Absence seizures in children: Clinical and electroencephalographic features. Ann Neurol 1987;21:268–273.

6. Deonna, TW. Acquired epileptiform aphasia in children (Landau-Kleffner syndrome). J Clin Neurophysiol 1991;8:288–298.

7. Hirsch, E, Marescaux, C, Maquet, P, Metz-Lutz, N, Kiesmann, M, Salmon, E, et al. Landau-Kleffner syndrome: A clinical and EEG study of five cases. Epilepsia 1990;31:756–767.

8. Tassinari, CA, Rubboli, G, Volpi, L, Meletti, S, d'Orsi, G, Franca, M, et al. Encephalopathy with electrical status epilepticus during slow sleep or ESES syndrome including the acquired aphasia. Clin Neurophysiol 2000;111:S94–S102.

CHAPTER 13

Non-epileptiform EEG abnormalities

In a very practical sense, the electroencephalogram (EEG) can be divided into two groups: normal and abnormal. There are two broad groups of abnormal EEGs: epileptiform and non-epileptiform. We have discussed epileptiform abnormalities in the previous chapters and this chapter focuses on non-epileptiform EEG abnormalities. Slowing, attenuation of activity, increase of activity, and coma/encephalopathy patterns are the main non-epileptiform abnormalities (Figure 13.1). Coma patterns are described in a subsequent chapter and we will focus on other non-epileptiform abnormalities here.

SLOWING

When describing slowing, one has to pay attention to:

1. The distribution: Posterior background, focal, multifocal, regional, hemispheric, generalized. This is the key element in describing the slow activity.

2. Amplitude.

3. Frequency: Theta and delta.

4. Persistence of slowing: Intermittent versus continuous.

5. Rhythmicity: Slow waves of the same duration (frequency) occurring in runs are considered rhythmic.

6. Regularity: Slow waves of the same morphology occurring in runs are considered regular (monomorphic). When the morphology is variable, it is called irregular (polymorphic).

7. Reactivity: Variability of slowing with stimuli or the state of vigilance is referred to as reactivity.

Posterior background slowing

The slowing of the posterior dominant rhythm indicates encephalopathy or diffuse cerebral dysfunction, including dementias (Figure 13.2). Loss of reactivity, the degree of slowing, and persistence of slowing (continuous rather than intermittent) tend to correlate with the severity of the underlying process. Unilateral posterior background slowing usually indicates the ipsilateral structural abnormality of dysfunction. One must always carefully look for the physiological causes of background slowing, such as drowsiness. It must also not be forgotten that the posterior background frequency is age-dependent. In general, in an adult, <8 Hz should be considered abnormal. It is also useful to study serial EEGs when available. Progressive background slowing, even if the frequency remains above 8 Hz, indicates an evolving abnormality of the brain. Alpha rhythm is thought to be cortical in origin and modulated by thalamocortical pathways. Disruption of these connections is likely to cause background slowing. It should be emphasized that posterior background slowing may be normal in some situations, e.g., slow alpha variant and posterior slow wave of youth variant.

 DOI: 10.1201/9781003353713-16

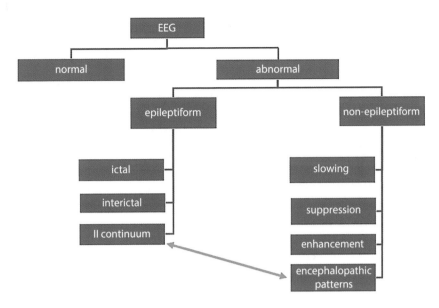

Figure 13.1   Classification of EEG abnormalities.

Focal/multifocal/regional/hemispheric slowing

Focal refers to a small area of the brain whereas "regional" indicates the involvement of a particular lobe (e.g., frontal, temporal). Multifocal means three or more spatially separated multiple areas (foci) and multiregional refers to the involvement of three or more lobes. Any slow activity spread across an entire hemisphere is identified as lateralized or hemispheric slowing.

Animal studies have shown that pure cortical lesions give rise to EEG amplitude attenuation rather than slowing. However, subcortical white matter lesions result in irregular delta slowing recorded from the overlying cortex. Thalamic lesions also cause focal or hemispheric delta slowing, whereas bilateral hypothalamic and upper mid-brain lesions produce bilateral slowing.[1] These data suggest that the deafferentation of the cortex from the subcortical structures is responsible for slowing.

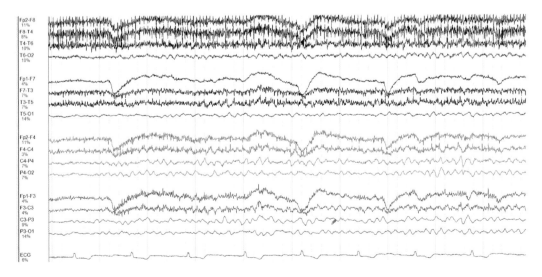

Figure 13.2   Slowing of the posterior dominant rhythm. This EEG was recorded from a patient with Alzheimer's dementia. Note the posterior dominant rhythm consists of 6.5 Hz theta activity.

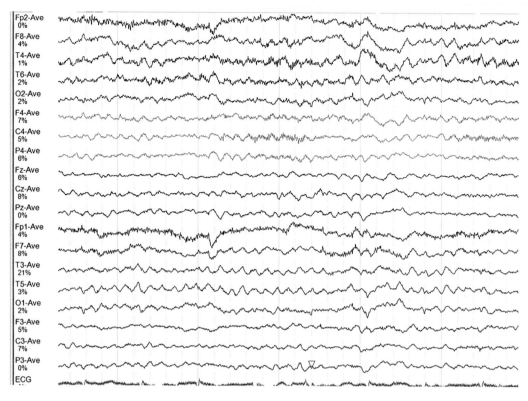

Figure 13.3 **Focal slowing.** Note theta and delta slowing the F8T4 electrodes in this patient with right temporal lobe epilepsy.

Non-generalized slowing is caused by underlying structural abnormalities or dysfunction (Figure 13.3). Abnormal background activity, the persistence of slowing (continuous rather than intermittent), and loss of reactivity are the best indicators of the severity of the underlying etiology of focal slowing, whilst topography, amplitude, and frequency do not appear to be important.[2] Irregular and arrhythmic (polymorphic) slowing usually indicates an underlying structural abnormality, whereas rhythmic slowing is more in favor of electrophysiological dysfunction. Polymorphic and continuous focal delta slowing is highly suggestive of an underlying structural abnormality. Postictal focal slowing has a good lateralizing value for the seizure focus. It should be remembered that focal slowing is not always abnormal. Temporal theta slowing is a normal finding in people older than 50 years of age. Normal variants of focal slowing (e.g., rhythmic mid-temporal theta of drowsiness) have been discussed in Chapter 8.

Generalized slowing

Generalized slowing indicates diffuse cerebral dysfunction, including encephalopathies of varying etiology (Figure 13.4). Bilateral mid-brain lesions involving the reticular formation and bilateral hypothalamic lesions also result in generalized slowing. Generalized slowing may be arrhythmic or rhythmic as in generalized rhythmic delta activity (GRDA). Frontal intermittent rhythmic delta (FIRDA) is a particular type of slowing included under the umbrella of GRDA (Figure 13.5). As the acronym suggests, FIRDA is characterized by bifrontal (or occasionally unilateral) synchronous runs of 1.5 to 2.5 Hz and regular and rhythmic sinusoidal or sawtooth waves.[3] Symmetrical FIRDA is usually seen in encephalopathies, whilst asymmetric FIRDA is caused by underlying structural abnormalities.[4] Asymmetric FIRDA should, however, be classified as a focal abnormality, whereas symmetric FIRDA is included as a form of generalized slowing. FIRDA can occasionally be seen in healthy individuals during hyperventilation.[4] FIRDA occurs predominantly during drowsiness and sleep.[4] Generalized slowing is a normal finding during sleep and hyperventilation.

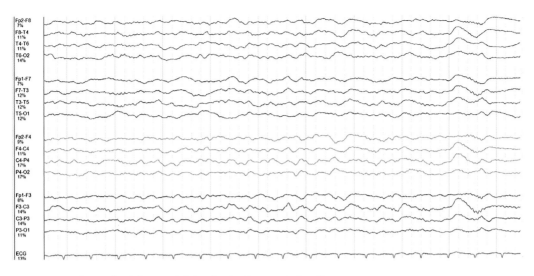

Figure 13.4 Generalized theta and delta slowing in encephalopathy.

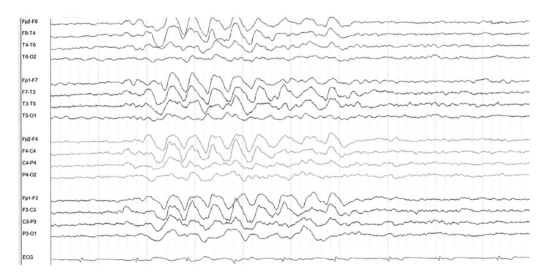

Figure 13.5 Frontal intermittent rhythmic delta activity.

ATTENUATION OF ACTIVITY

Focal attenuation

As previously discussed, attenuation refers to amplitude decrease. Attenuation is usually accompanied by frequency changes as well. There are three main reasons for attenuation:

1. *Technical:* When comparing homologous electrodes, the inter-electrode distance is an important consideration and an error in measurement in placing the electrodes by the technologist can result in an apparent asymmetry in amplitudes giving the impression of suppression. As we have already discussed in Chapter 3, the EEG waveform amplitude reflects the voltage difference between two electrodes. If the inter-electrode distance is smaller than the homologous pair, the amplitude is displayed lower than the homologous pair, giving the false impression of suppression.

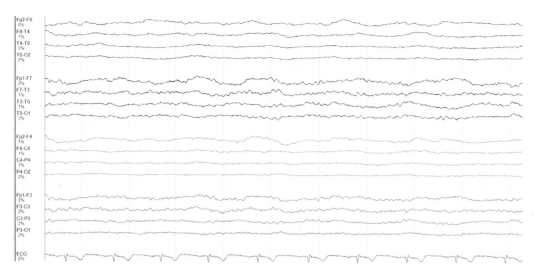

Figure 13.6 Attenuation of EEG activity. The CT brain scan of the patient shows a large right-sided sub-arachnoid hemorrhage and brain swelling. There is also evidence of scalp edema on the right. The attenuation of EEG waveforms on the right hemisphere here is multifactorial: Increased distance from the cortex to the electrode and hemispheric dysfunction.

2. *Focal cortical lesions or dysfunction:* Cortical lesions give rise to attenuation whilst subcortical involvement results in slowing. Similarly, focal (hemispheric) attenuation of beta activity[5] or sleep patterns/waveforms[6] indicates underlying dysfunction or structural abnormality. Sometimes, beta activity can be augmented (increased amplitude) ipsilateral to the lesion, particularly in chronic lesions.[5] Hence, one needs to be careful about the lateralizing value of the asymmetry. Ipsilateral attenuation and the slowing of posterior dominant rhythm occur due to acute or progressive focal lesions. It has a better lateralizing value than a localizing value. Occasionally, alpha amplitude may increase ipsilaterally with chronic lesions (e.g., infarct) and slow-growing tumors. However, in those cases, the posterior dominant rhythm tends to be slower and less reactive on the same side.[7]

3. *Increased distance from the cerebral cortex to the recording electrode:* This could be due to lesions involving any layer; scalp (edema, hematoma), extradural hematoma, subdural hematoma, and dural tumors (Figure 13.6).

Generalized attenuation

Generalized attenuation indicates diffuse cortical dysfunction as seen in hypoxic ischemic encephalopathy. When the amplitudes are <10 microvolts, the term "suppression" is used. The same changes can be caused by anesthetic medications. Good examples are suppression and burst suppression due to propofol and barbiturates. Some healthy individuals have low-amplitude EEGs and generalized attenuation does not always indicate a pathological cause.

INCREASE IN ACTIVITY

Focal increase

The most common cause of the focal increase is skull defects giving rise to breach rhythm. We have discussed breach rhythm in detail in a previous chapter. Occasionally, focal lesions may result in increased focal activity as discussed in the previous section.

Generalized increase

Excessive beta activity is usually caused by drugs such as benzodiazepines, barbiturates, and neuroleptics.

ABNORMALITIES IN ENCEPHALOPATHY AND COMA

This group consists of burst suppression, electrocerebral inactivity, periodic discharges, triphasic waves, and coma patterns (alpha, beta, theta/delta, spindle). These non-epileptiform abnormalities will be discussed in Chapter 17.

References

1. Gloor, P, Ball, G, Schaul, N. Brain lesions that produce delta waves in the EEG. Neurology 1977;27: 326–333.

2. Schaul, N, Green, L, Peyster, R, Gotman, J. Structural determinants of electroencephalographic findings in acute hemispheric lesions. Ann Neurol 1986;20:703–711.

3. Kane, N, Acharya, J, Benickzy, S, Caboclo, L, Finnigan, S, Kaplan, PW, et al. A revised glossary of terms most commonly used by clinical electroencephalographers and updated proposal for the report format of the EEG findings. Revision 2017. Clin Neurophysiol Pract 2017;2:170–185.

4. Accolla, EA, Kaplan, PW, Maeder-Ingvar, M, Jukopila, S, Rossetti, AO. Clinical correlates of frontal intermittent rhythmic delta activity (FIRDA). Clin Neurophysiol 2011;122:27–31.

5. Green, RL, Wilson, WP. Asymmetries of beta activity in epilepsy, brain tumor, and cerebrovascular disease. Electroencephalogr Clin Neurophysiol 1961;13:75–78.

6. Daly, DD. The effect of sleep upon the electroencephalogram in patients with brain tumors. Electroencephalogr Clin Neurophysiol 1968;25:521–529.

7. Markand, ON. Alpha rhythms. J Clin Neurophysiol 1990;7:163–190.

CHAPTER 14

EEG in dementia

Many neurological conditions are grouped under the umbrella of dementing disorders. This spectrum includes Alzheimer's disease (AD), vascular dementia (VD), dementia with Lewy bodies (DLB), fronto-temporal dementia (FTD), and Creutzfeldt-Jacob disease (CJD). Most abnormalities seen in dementias are non-specific to the etiology except for the more striking changes in CJD. It is also important to differentiate from normal electroencephalogram (EEG) changes with aging. Though some slowing of posterior dominant rhythm (PDR) is expected with aging, slowing of <8 Hz is unusual and is considered abnormal.[1] Temporal slow waves can be a normal finding in healthy individuals older than 60 years of age. These slow waves tend to be attenuated by eye-opening and enhanced by drowsiness and hyperventilation. They usually occur intermittently as single waves with rounded morphology or pairs with amplitudes <70 microvolts. The frequency is usually in the theta range or occasionally delta, but the slowing lasts for <1% of the recording.[2]

ALZHEIMER'S DISEASE

In the early stages of AD, quantitative EEG may show an increase in slow activity, but the visual analysis is usually normal. As the condition advances, the EEG changes become more apparent. The slowing of the PDR to the theta and delta ranges is an early change. Generalized slowing appears with a fronto-temporal emphasis. Approximately 10–20% of patients experience unprovoked seizures. Epileptiform discharges, typically focal, are seen among 62% of patients with seizures and 6% without a history of seizures. Those with seizures as well as subclinical epileptiform discharges experience cognitive decline earlier than others.[3] Generalized triphasic waves with occipital emphasis can be seen in a minority of patients.[4]

DEMENTIA WITH LEWY BODIES

The vast majority of studies have been conducted in this field with quantitative EEG. However, visual analysis of the EEG can also be helpful. Slowing, both generalized and focal, has been reported. Slowing of the PDR and focal temporal slow waves in DLB have been found to be more marked than in AD.[5] Some case studies have reported triphasic waves and frontal intermittent rhythmic delta activity (FIRDA).[6] In pathologically confirmed DLB, the seizure occurrence has been reported to be around 4%.[7]

CREUTZFELDT-JACOB DISEASE (CJD)

CJD is a relentlessly progressive and fatal prion disease characterized by rapidly progressive dementia and other neurological manifestations including myoclonus and seizures. The EEG plays a vital role in establishing the diagnosis. The changes depend on the disease stage. Stage I is characterized by neuropsychiatric symptoms accompanied by minor or no signs. A distinct neurological

 DOI: 10.1201/9781003353713-17

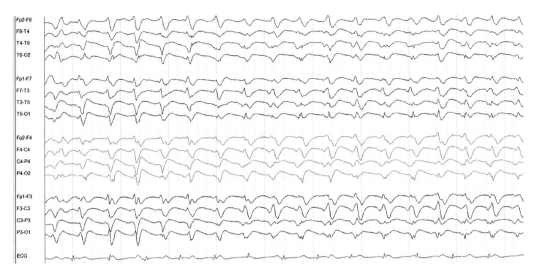

Figure 14.1 Typical EEG changes of generalized periodic discharges of triphasic morphology in Creutzfeldt-Jakob disease.

syndrome is seen in stage II and myoclonus may emerge in this stage. Stage III is the terminal phase, characterized by severe myoclonus, rapidly progressive dementia, and akinetic mutism leading to death.[8] In the early stages, the EEG changes are non-specific and include slowing of PDR, generalized slowing, and occasionally focal slowing. In stage II, generalized slowing is the main EEG abnormality, though periodic and non-periodic triphasic waves are seen occasionally.[9] Periodic discharges of triphasic morphology is the EEG hallmark of CJD seen in stage III; however, some patients demonstrate non-periodic triphasic waves during this stage.[9] FIRDA can also be seen during stage III.[9]

Generalized periodic discharges demonstrate certain characteristics. They typically have a triphasic morphology, 200–500 milliseconds in duration and 300 microvolts in amplitude, recurring at a frequency of 1 Hz (range 0.5–2 Hz) (Figure 14.1). Occasionally, periodic discharges can be unilateral and asymmetric, whilst some complexes demonstrate an anterior-posterior lag (Figure 14.2).[9]

Typically, the amplitude maximum of the discharges is seen over the fronto-precentral midline. Usually, periodic complexes demonstrate reactivity with attenuation during sleep and drowsiness.

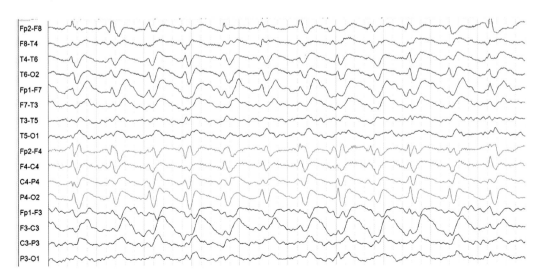

Figure 14.2 Lateralized periodic discharges of triphasic morphology in Creutzfeldt-Jakob disease.

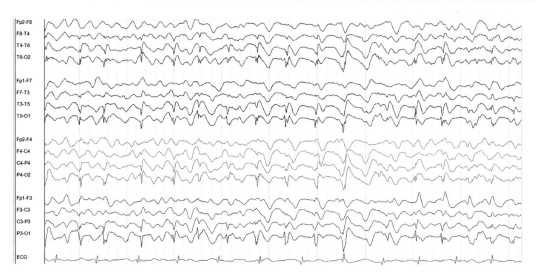

Figure 14.3   EEG of the Heidenhain variant of Creutzfeldt-Jakob disease showing posterior dominant periodic discharges.

Similarly, periodic complexes may appear with external stimuli including intermittent photic stimulation. Myoclonic jerks may appear with periodic discharges, but this relationship is not always consistent.[10] The periodic complexes tend to have a more posterior emphasis in the Heidenhain variant of CJD (Figure 14.3).

With the advancing disease process, the amplitude and the frequency of periodic discharges gradually decrease, completely disappearing in the terminal stages. Finally, the EEG shows attenuation of EEG activity with occasional bursts of slowing. Due to this progressive nature of EEG changes, it is useful to repeat the EEG in suspected cases of CJD when the first EEG shows non-diagnostic features (Figure 14.4a & b).

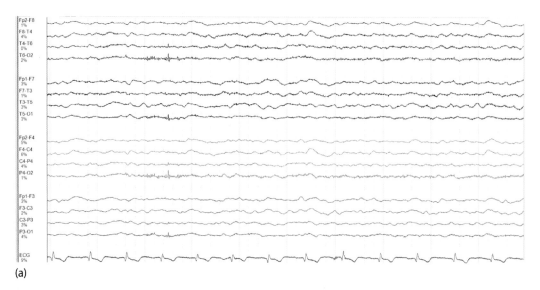

(a)

Figure 14.4   The value of repeating the EEG in Creutzfeldt-Jakob disease. (a) This first EEG shows generalized slowing in a patient who presented with rapidly progressive dementia. (b) The next EEG, one week later, shows generalized periodic discharges highly suggestive of Creutzfeldt-Jakob disease. The diagnosis of Creutzfeldt-Jakob disease was eventually confirmed with cerebrospinal fluid testing and typical MRI findings. *(Continued)*

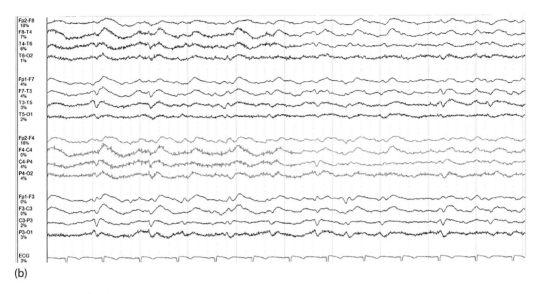

(b)

Figure 14.4 *(Continued)*

References

1. Katz, RI, Horowitz, GR. Electroencephalogram in the septuagenarian: Studies in a normal geriatric population. J Am Geriatr Soc 1982;30(4):273–275.

2. Klass, DW, Brenner, RP. Electroencephalography of the elderly. J Clin Neurophysiol 1995;12(2):116–131.

3. Vossel, KA, Beagle, AJ, Rabinovici, GD, Shu, H, Lee, SE, Naasan, G, et al. Seizures and epileptiform activity in the early stages of Alzheimer disease JAMA Neurol. 2013;70(9):1158–1166.

4. Primavera, A, Traverso, F. Triphasic waves in Alzheimer's disease. Acta Neurol Belg 1990;90(5):274–281.

5. Briel, RC, McKeith, IG, Barker, WA, Hewitt, Y, Perry, RH, Ince, PG, et al. EEG findings in dementia with Lewy bodies and Alzheimer's disease J Neurol Neurosurg Psychiatry. 1999 Mar;66(3):401–403.

6. Chatzikonstantinou, S, McKenna, J, Karantali, E, Petridis, F, Kazis, D, Mavroudis, I. Electroencephalogram in dementia with Lewy bodies: A systematic review Aging Clin Exp Res. 2020 May 7.

7. Marawar, R, Wakim, N, Albin, RL, Dodge, H. Seizure occurrence and related mortality in dementia with Lewy bodies. Epilepsy Behav 2020 Jul 18;111:107311.

8. Roos, R, Gajdusek, DC, Gibbs, CJ. Jr. The clinical characteristics of transmissible Creutzfeldt-Jakob disease. Brain 1973;96(1):1–20.

9. Ayyappan, S, Seneviratne, U. Electroencephalographic changes in sporadic Creutzfeldt-Jakob disease and correlation with clinical stages: A retrospective analysis. J Clin Neurophysiol 2014;31(6):586–593.

10. Burger, LJ, Rowan, AJ, Goldensohn, ES. Creutzfeldt-Jakob disease: An Electroencephalographic Study. Arch Neurol 1972;26(5):428–433.

Critical care EEG

CHAPTER 15

Ictal-interictal continuum

In Chapter 9, the concept of the ictal-interictal continuum (IIC) was introduced as the border zone between interictal/encephalopathic and ictal epileptiform abnormalities. The details of IIC are best discussed in the last section of this book dedicated to critical care EEG, including non-convulsive status epilepticus, encephalopathy, and coma, as these patterns are typically seen in critically ill patients with overlapping features.

The term IIC was first introduced in 1996, conceptualizing the generation of periodic lateralized epileptiform discharges (now called "lateralized periodic discharges").[1] Subsequently, it became clear there are several rhythmic and periodic patterns seen in the setting of critically ill patients, and the application of the term IIC was expanded to encompass all such patterns. The American Clinical Neurophysiology Society (ACNS) published the descriptive terminology to be applied in this entity.[2] These patterns are typically seen in critically ill patients in coma being treated in the intensive care unit. Though some patterns may look highly suspicious for electrographic seizures, they do not fulfill the criteria of an ictal rhythm.[3] Hence, IIC deserves discussion as a discrete entity and should be distinguished from non-convulsive status epilepticus and encephalopathic patterns seen in critically ill patients.

The ACNS critical care EEG terminology forms the foundation of identifying and describing IIC. To describe rhythmic and periodic patterns of IIC, the terminology combines two main items and a set of modifiers, as shown in Table 15.1.[2] It is important to emphasize that ACNS terminology is not exclusive to IIC and covers the entire spectrum of EEG abnormalities encountered in the critical care setting.

MAIN TERM #1

Generalized patterns refer to bilateral, symmetric, and synchronous waveforms, including bifrontal activity. Generalized patterns can be frontally, occipitally, or midline predominant. When the activity is confined to a single hemisphere, which may be focal, regional, or hemispheric, the term "lateralized" is applied. Bilateral and synchronous, but asymmetric waveforms are also considered lateralized ("lateralized-bilateral asymmetric"). Bilateral independent patterns refer to two asynchronous and independent lateralized activities. Three or more lateralized and independent patterns, seen in both hemispheres, are termed "multifocal".[2]

MAIN TERM #2

The main elements of periodic discharges are the discharge and the inter-discharge interval. Discharges are defined as any waveform with (1) three or fewer phases lasting 0.5 seconds or more or (2) duration of <0.5 seconds irrespective of the phases. If the waveform has four or more phases and lasts 0.5 seconds or more, the term "burst" is applied. From the definition, it should be

DOI: 10.1201/9781003353713-19

Table 15.1 Critical care EEG terminology for rhythmic and periodic patterns

Main term 1	Main term 2	Modifiers

1 Generalized
2 Lateralized
3 Bilateral independent
4 Unilateral independent
5 Multifocal
	1 Periodic discharges
	2 Rhythmic delta activity
	3 Spike and wave, polyspike and wave, or sharp and wave
		Major modifiers
		1 Prevalence
		2 Duration
		3 Frequency
		4 Number of phases
		5 Sharpness
		6 Amplitude of the waveforms
		7 Stimulus-induced or stimulus-terminated
		8 Evolution, fluctuation, or static
		9 "Plus" features
		  • Superimposed fast (+F)
		  • Superimposed rhythmic (+R)
		  • Superimposed sharp waves/spikes/
		    sharply contoured waves (+S)
		  • Superimposed fast and rhythmic
		    activity with periodic discharges (+FR)
		  • Superimposed fast and sharp activity
		    with rhythmic delta activity (+FS)
		
		Minor modifiers
		1 Sudden onset or gradual onset
		2 Triphasic morphology
		3 Anterior-posterior, posterior-anterior lag,
		  or no lag
		4 Polarity- positive/negative/dipole/unclear

noted that discharges are not synonymous with the term "epileptiform discharges" used in EEG reporting. According to the critical care EEG terminology, even triphasic waves are classified as "discharges." To qualify as periodic, the inter-discharge interval can only vary by <50% between the consecutive cycles in >50% of cycle pairs of the EEG record. Rhythmic delta activity refers to slow waves of ≤4 Hz repeating with uniform morphology and duration. The cycle duration can only vary by <50% in the majority (>50%) of pairs, according to the ACNS criteria. Additionally, to be defined as periodic or rhythmic, the pattern should persist for at least six cycles.[2]

MODIFIERS

There are numerous modifiers used in the description of critical care EEGs as highlighted in Table 15.1. However, the most important modifiers in IIC are "plus" features and stimulus-induced changes. These are additional features superimposed on an existing pattern shifting the balance towards being more "ictal-like." There are four important plus features: (1) superimposed fast activity (+F) coexisting with periodic discharges and rhythmic delta activity, (2) superimposed rhythmic activity (+R) occurring with periodic discharges (Figure 15.1), (3) superimposed sharp waves or spikes (+S) overlapping with rhythmic delta activity, and (4) combinations (+FR) with periodic discharges and +FS with rhythmic delta activity. Stimulus-induced patterns are triggered by alerting stimuli (auditory, tactile, pain, etc.) and are reproducible.[2] The stimulus-induced pattern can be rhythmic delta activity, periodic discharges, BIRDs, or seizures.

PATTERNS OF ICTAL-INTERICTAL CONTINUUM

The patterns of IIC lie along a spectrum in which some patterns are closer to the "ictal" end and the others gravitate toward the "non-ictal" (encephalopathy) pole or in the middle. Rhythmicity and periodicity with or without plus features, as defined by the critical care EEG terminology, are the cornerstones in recognizing IIC. These patterns can be potentially ictal, but do not fulfill the criteria for electrographic seizures or electrographic status epilepticus.

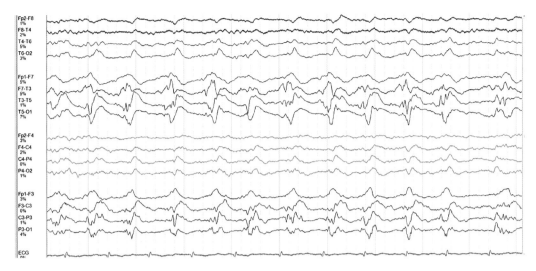

Figure 15.1   Lateralized (bilateral asymmetric) periodic discharges with plus features – superimposed rhythmic and fast activities.

Lateralized/Bilateral independent/Multifocal periodic discharges

The definitions of lateralized periodic discharges (LDP), bilateral independent periodic discharges (BIPD), and multifocal periodic discharges (MFPD) have been explained under main terms 1 and 2 of the ACNS terminology (Figures 15.2 and 15.3). Any type of periodic discharges of (a) >1 to ≤2.5 Hz lasting 10 seconds or more, and (b) ≥0.5 to ≤1 Hz with plus features or fluctuation lasting 10 seconds or more are typically included in the IIC. Any PDs of >2.5 Hz lasting 10 or more seconds would satisfy the definition of an electrographic seizure.

These patterns are closer to the "ictal" pole of the IIC spectrum. The presence of plus features and higher frequencies (>2 Hz) make the patterns more likely to be ictal.[4] The old terminology for LPD is periodic lateralized epileptiform discharges (PLEDs), the use of which is discouraged in the current nomenclature. These patterns are usually seen in the setting of acute brain insults ranging from infections (e.g., encephalitis), vasculitis, inflammation, and stroke to neoplasia. Additionally, these patterns are often encountered in close association with seizures and non-convulsive status epilepticus (NCSE) confirming the "ictal" nature of this pattern (Figure 15.4a & b). This will be further discussed in Chapter 16.

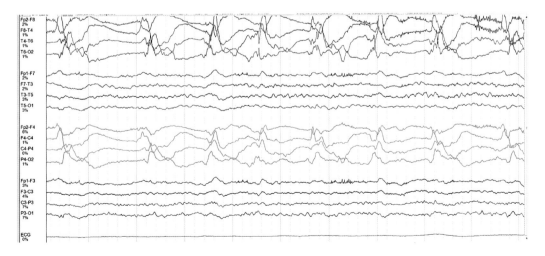

Figure 15.2   Lateralized periodic discharges involving the right cerebral hemisphere.

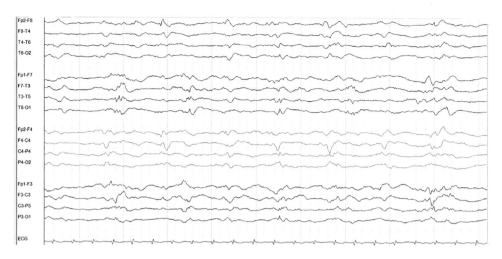

Figure 15.3   Bilateral independent periodic discharges.

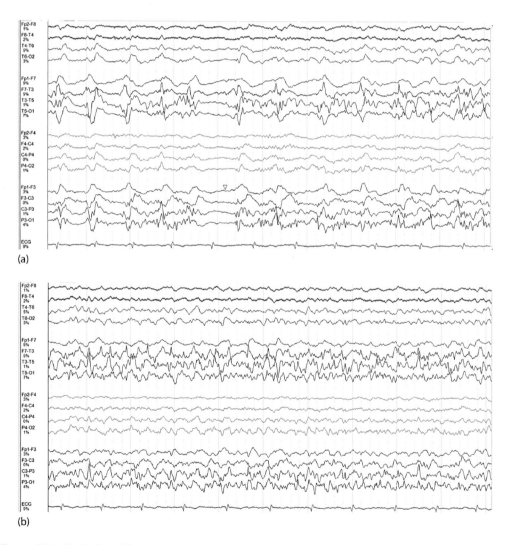

(a)

(b)

Figure 15.4   Evolution of lateralized periodic discharges into an ictal rhythm in non-convulsive status epilepticus. (a) The first 4 seconds of the epoch demonstrates LPD+, which evolves into an ictal rhythm in the second half of the epoch. (b) Further evolution of the ictal rhythm.

Generalized periodic discharges

Often encountered in toxic and metabolic encephalopathies, generalized periodic discharges (GPD) tend to lie in the middle of the IIC spectrum (Figure 15.5a & b). However, faster frequencies (>2 Hz) and the presence of plus features shift this pattern toward the "ictal" pole. Periodic triphasic waves seen in renal and liver failure are a classic example of GPD. The notion that periodic triphasic waves are synonymous with toxic/metabolic encephalopathy is a myth and GPD of triphasic morphology has been described in association with seizures and NCSE.[5]

Lateralized rhythmic delta activity

Lateralized rhythmic delta activity (LRDA) is an IIC pattern predictive of seizures similar to LPD (Figure 15.6). LRDA of >1 Hz with plus features or fluctuation lasting 10 or more seconds is considered to be IIC.

One study demonstrated that 63% of patients with LRDA went on to experience seizures during the acute illness comparable to 57% in LPD.[6] Again, the presence of plus features and faster frequencies (>2 Hz) increase the likelihood of "ictal" transformation.

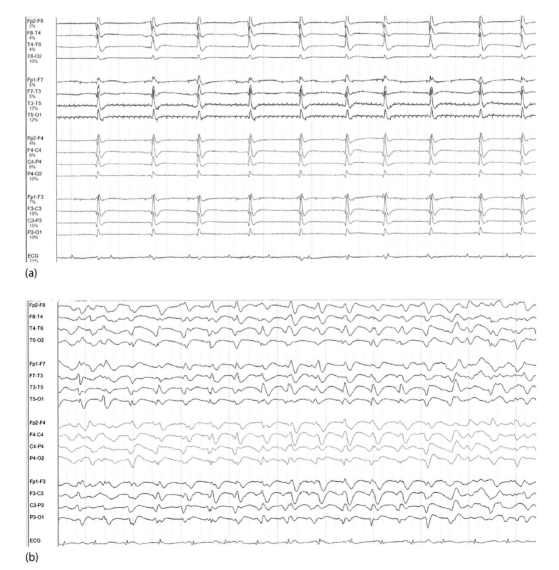

(a)

(b)

Figure 15.5 Generalized periodic discharges with sharp wave morphology (a) and triphasic wave morphology (b).

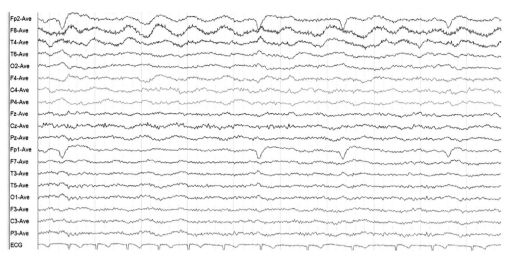

Figure 15.6   Lateralized rhythmic delta activity.

Generalized rhythmic delta activity

Generalized rhythmic delta activity (GRDA) is mostly an encephalopathic pattern with no significant association with seizures (Figure 15.7).[7]

Stimulus-induced rhythmic, periodic, or ictal discharges

Stimulus-induced rhythmic, periodic, or ictal discharges (SIRPIDs) are seen in the critical care EEGs of patients with varying etiologies such as toxic/metabolic encephalopathy, cerebral trauma, intracranial hemorrhage, and hypoxic brain injury.[8] SIRPIDs are defined as periodic, rhythmic, or evolving ictal discharges consistently triggered by alerting stimuli (Figure 15.8a & b).[9] A study found SIRPIDs to be significantly associated with hypoxic brain injury and electrographic seizures.[8] Stimulus-induced seizures are included under the umbrella of SIRPIDs, but not considered to be in the spectrum if IIC.

Brief potentially ictal rhythmic discharges

Brief potentially ictal rhythmic discharges or B(I)RDs are defined as focal or generalized sharply contoured rhythmic activity of >4 Hz with or without evolution lasting ≥0.5 to <10 seconds and not

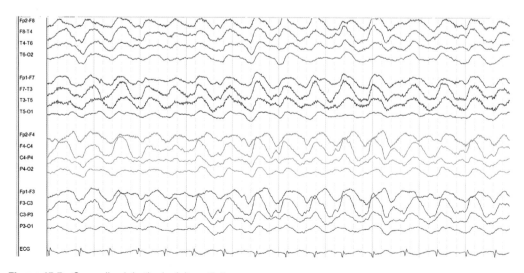

Figure 15.7   Generalized rhythmic delta activity.

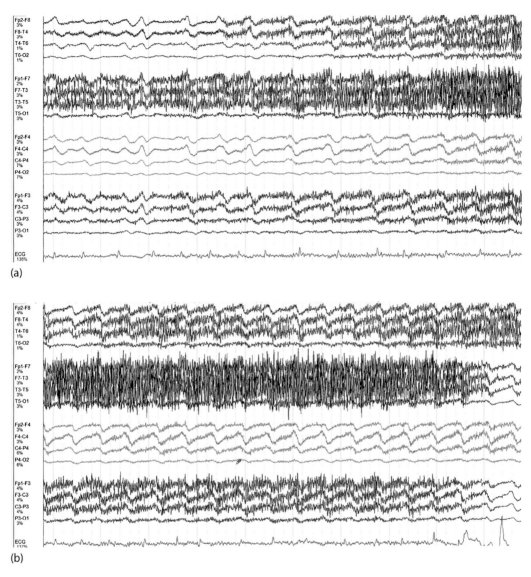

Figure 15.8 Stimulus-induced rhythmic, periodic, or ictal discharges (SIRPIDs). EEG recorded from an unconscious patient in the intensive care unit. (a) Suctioning of secretion by a nurse in the third second of this EEG epoch triggers a run of generalized rhythmic activity. (b) Continuation of rhythmic activity with no evolution.

associated with any clinical correlates or burst suppression/attenuation (Figure 15.9).[10] The vast majority of patients with B(I)RDs have an underlying structural brain abnormality, but it can also be seen in hypoxic brain injury.[11] B(I)RDs are associated with a 75% prevalence of seizures in critically ill patients.[11]

PREDICTION OF SEIZURE RISK

The main dilemma for the clinician when encountered with IIC is the estimation of seizure risk. The 2HELPS2B score has been proposed to fill this void.[12] This tool takes into consideration the ictal potential of different IIC patterns. Higher frequencies (>2 Hz) and plus features score extra points. Table 15.2 highlights the different components of the tool.[12]

The probable risk of seizures increases with the score; 5% for score 0, 12% for 1, 27% for 2, 50% for 3, 73% for 4, 88% for 5, and >95% for >6.[12]

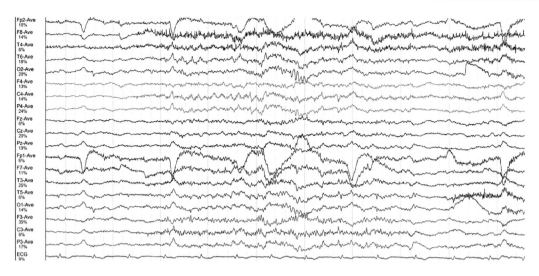

Figure 15.9   Brief potentially ictal rhythmic discharges.

Table 15.2   Components of the 2HELPS2B tool

	EEG abnormality	Score
2H	**>2 Hz** frequency for any periodic or rhythmic pattern (GRDA/LRDA/BIPD/GPD/LPD)	1
E	**E**pileptiform discharges-sporadic	1
L	**L**ateralized rhythms (LPD/LRDA/BIPD)	1
P	**P**lus features (GRDA/LRDA/BIPD/LPD/GPD with superimposed rhythmic, fast or sharp activity)	1
S	**S**eizure history – any (acute or remote)	1
2B	**B**(I)RDS	2

HOW TO TREAT ICTAL-INTERICTAL CONTINUUM

The management of IIC is challenging. There are no universally accepted guidelines. Experts have published treatment algorithms.[4,13] Essentially, the presence of higher frequencies (>2 Hz) and plus features favor a trial of antiseizure medications. The 2HELPS2B score can be used as an adjunct in the process of this decision making.

References

1. Pohlmann-Eden, B, Hoch, DB, Cochius, JI, Chiappa, KH. Periodic lateralized epileptiform discharges–a critical review. J Clin Neurophysiol 1996;13(6):519–530.

2. Hirsch, LJ, Fong, MWK, Leitinger, M, et al. American Clinical Neurophysiology Society's standardized critical care EEG terminology: 2021 Version. J Clin Neurophysiol 2021;38(1):1–29.

3. Chong, DJ, Hirsch, LJ. Which EEG patterns warrant treatment in the critically ill? Reviewing the evidence for treatment of periodic epileptiform discharges and related patterns. J Clin Neurophysiol 2005;22(2):79–91.

4. Rodriguez, V, Rodden, MF, LaRoche, SM. Ictal-interictal continuum: A proposed treatment algorithm. Clin Neurophysiol 2016;127(4):2056–2064.

5. Foreman, B, Claassen, J, Abou Khaled, K, Jirsch, J, Alschuler, DM, Wittman, J, et al. Generalized periodic discharges in the critically ill a case-control study of 200 patients. Neurology 2012;79(19):1951–1960.

6. Gaspard, N, Manganas, L, Rampal, N, Petroff, OAC, Hirsch, LJ. Similarity of lateralized rhythmic delta activity to periodic lateralized epileptiform discharges in critically ill patients. JAMA Neurology 2013;70(10):1288–1295.

7. Rodriguez Ruiz, A, Vlachy, J, Lee, JW, Gilmore, EJ, Ayer, T, Haider, HA, et al. Association of periodic and rhythmic electroencephalographic patterns with seizures in critically ill patients JAMA Neurol. 2017 Feb 1;74(2):181–188.

8. Braksick, SA, Burkholder, DB, Tsetsou, S, Martineau, L, Mandrekar, J, Rossetti, AO, et al. Associated factors and prognostic implications of stimulus-induced rhythmic, periodic, or ictal discharges JAMA Neurol. 2016 May 1;73(5):585–590.

9. Hirsch, LJ, Claassen, J, Mayer, SA, Emerson, RG. Stimulus-induced rhythmic, periodic, or ictal discharges (SIRPIDs): A common EEG phenomenon in the critically ill. Epilepsia 2004;45(2):109–123.

10. Yoo, JY, Marcuse, LV, Fields, MC, Rosengard, JL, Traversa, MV, Gaspard, N, et al. Brief potentially ictal rhythmic discharges [B(I)RDs] in noncritically ill adults J Clin Neurophysiol. 2017 May;34(3):222–229.

11. Yoo, JY, Rampal, N, Petroff, OA, Hirsch, LJ, Gaspard, N. Brief potentially ictal rhythmic discharges in critically ill adults. JAMA Neurol 2014;71(4):454–462.

12. Struck, AF, Ustun, B, Ruiz, AR, Lee, JW, LaRoche, SM, Hirsch, LJ, et al. Association of an electroencephalography-based risk score with seizure probability in hospitalized patients JAMA Neurol. 2017 Dec 1;74(12):1419–1424.

13. Claassen, J. How I treat patients with EEG patterns on the ictal-interictal continuum in the neuro ICU. Neurocrit Care 2009;11(3):437–444.

CHAPTER 16

Non-convulsive status epilepticus

WHAT IS STATUS EPILEPTICUS

To lay the foundation to discuss non-convulsive status epilepticus (NCSE), we should first understand the definition of status epilepticus (SE). SE is diagnosed when a seizure is sufficiently prolonged to "produce an enduring epileptic condition."[1] In the current terminology, there are two critical time points concerning SE: t1, which indicates abnormally prolonged seizure with no possibility of spontaneous termination; and t2, beyond which point long-term consequences such as neuronal injury and death are likely to occur.[1] These time points vary depending on the seizure type. For example, in tonic-clonic SE, t1 is 5 minutes and t2 is 30 minutes, whilst for focal SE with impaired awareness, those time points are 10 and >60 minutes, respectively.[1]

CLASSIFICATION OF STATUS EPILEPTICUS

In the International League Against Epilepsy (ILAE) classification, there are two major groups of SE: with and without prominent motor symptoms. Convulsive, myoclonic, focal motor, tonic, and hyperkinetic seizure types are included under the umbrella of SE *with* motor features.[1]

Status epilepticus *without* prominent motor symptoms essentially comprises a spectrum of seizure types classified as non-convulsive status epilepticus.

Status epilepticus *with* prominent motor symptoms:

1. Convulsive (tonic-clonic) SE
   a. Generalized tonic-clonic SE
   b. Focal to bilateral tonic-clonic SE
   c. Unknown onset tonic-clonic SE
2. Myoclonic SE
3. Focal motor SE
4. Tonic SE
5. Hyperkinetic SE

Status epilepticus *without* prominent motor symptoms (NCSE):

1. NCSE with coma
2. NCSE without coma
   a. Generalized onset: Typical absence SE, atypical absence SE, myoclonic absence SE
   b. Focal onset: With impaired consciousness, without impaired consciousness, aphasic SE
   c. Unknown onset: Autonomic SE

DOI: 10.1201/9781003353713-20

ETIOLOGY OF NCSE

There is a wide spectrum of conditions, including both acute and chronic, giving rise to NCSE. The main chronic condition of interest is underlying epilepsy. Acute etiologies include critical illnesses in the ICU, traumatic brain injury, acute stroke, acute intracranial hemorrhage, encephalitis, hypoxic-ischemic brain injury, and drugs (including baclofen, lithium, and opioids). The incidence of NCSE and resultant mortality increases with age. Among the elderly, cerebrovascular disease, metabolic derangement, brain tumors, head injury, sepsis, and pre-existing epilepsy are among the most frequently reported etiologies.[2]

SYMPTOMS OF NCSE

Impaired consciousness

The reduced conscious state is a key feature in NCSE seen in more than 80% of cases, though some types present without any alteration of the sensorium.[3] The impairment in consciousness may range from subtle changes to deep coma. Reductions in consciousness can be due to NCSE, encephalopathy, or structural brain damage. In a patient with extensive brain injury and a localized seizure captured on the EEG, the reduced conscious state can be due to structural brain damage rather than the seizure. Hence, the clinical picture should be carefully interpreted in the context of history, EEG, and neuroimaging findings.

Speech disturbances

Speech disturbances are encountered in approximately 15% of cases diagnosed with NCSE.[3] The spectrum of speech disturbances is wide, ranging from speech arrest, dysphasia, alexia, and dysarthria to vocalization.

Cognitive and behavioral changes

Though one would expect to find cognitive deficits and behavioral changes depending on the brain regions involved, the studies are scant. Executive dysfunction, reduced working memory, agnosia, apraxia, and perseverative behaviors have been reported.[4,5]

Neuropsychiatric manifestations

Neuropsychiatric manifestations have been well described in NCSE. The spectrum of presentations includes hallucinations (visual, auditory, somatic), delusions, impulsive behavior, anxiety, agitation, delirium, catatonia, and affective symptoms.

Motor manifestations

By definition, NCSE is not accompanied by "prominent" motor symptoms. However subtle motor manifestations such as myoclonus, gaze deviation, and nystagmus are useful signs observed in NCSE.

Visual manifestations

NCSE arising from the primary visual cortex typically manifests with elementary visual hallucinations whereas more complex visual hallucinations and formed images are experienced by patients when the seizure activity involves more anterior occipitotemporal and occipito-parietal regions. Ictal blindness is a rare phenomenon.

Autonomic manifestations

Autonomic manifestations during NCSE are well recognized.[3] The spectrum includes pupillary abnormalities, flushing, sweating, hypertension, and cardiac arrhythmias. Panayiotopoulos syndrome is a childhood epilepsy syndrome that may present with NCSE characterized by prominent autonomic manifestations such as retching, vomiting, pallor, cyanosis, miosis, mydriasis, hypersalivation, and irregular breathing. Other ictal manifestations include eye deviation, visual hallucinations, and speech arrest.[6]

DIAGNOSTIC CRITERIA

According to the proposed "modified Salzburg Consensus Criteria," NCSE is diagnosed based on the combination of clinical and EEG criteria.[7]

Clinical criteria

1. Transition from the baseline to suspect NCSE within a period of minutes to hours.

2. Symptoms and signs last ≥10 minutes with no spontaneous recovery. Waxing and waning of symptoms are compatible with the diagnosis.

3. No alternative explanation for the EEG pattern based on neuroimaging.

4. No alternative explanation for the EEG pattern based on toxic/metabolic screening.

EEG criteria

Differentiating NCSE patterns from baseline abnormalities in those patients with a background epileptic encephalopathy can be challenging. Hence, there are additional requirements to diagnose NCSE in patients with epileptic encephalopathy.

Patients without known encephalopathy

The following EEG changes should last for ≥10 seconds. Criterion 1 or 2 should be satisfied to confirm NCSE.

1. A run of epileptiform discharges with a frequency of >2.5 Hz (Figure 16.1a & b)

2. If the ED frequency is ≤2.5 Hz or there is rhythmic delta/theta activity of >0.5 Hz, one of the following criteria should be fulfilled:

    a.   Spatio-temporal evolution (Figure 16.2a, b, & c).

    b.   Subtle clinical phenomena (subtle twitching in the peri-oral region/peri-orbital region/extremities with temporal relation to the EEG pattern.

    c.   Clinical and EEG improvement within 10 minutes following intravenous antiseizure medication administration. Patients must be tested before and after medication administration.

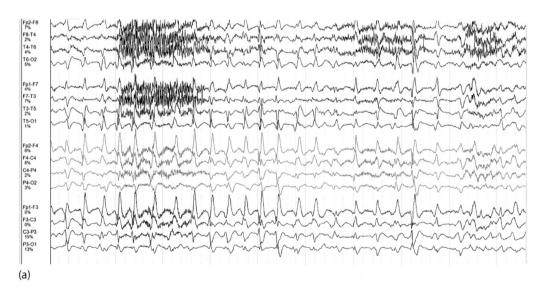

(a)

Figure 16.1   Non-convulsive status epilepticus. (a) A patient diagnosed with idiopathic generalized epilepsy had missed antiseizure medications for two days with an intercurrent chest infection and was admitted in an altered-conscious state. The EEG demonstrates generalized periodic discharges of 3 Hz, fulfilling the EEG criteria of NCSE. (b) The EEG is normalized 24 hours after treatment with intravenous sodium valproate. *(Continued)*

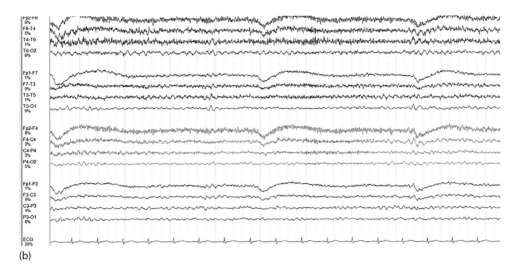

(b)

Figure 16.1   *(Continued)*

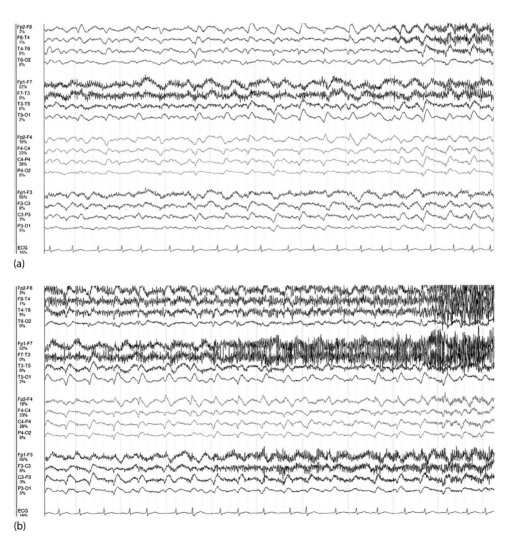

(a)

(b)

Figure 16.2   Non-convulsive status epilepticus diagnosed on the basis of spatio-temporal evolution.
(a) Generalized periodic discharges of 1.5 Hz. (b) & (c) Both figures illustrate the evolution in frequency and
morphology. *(Continued)*

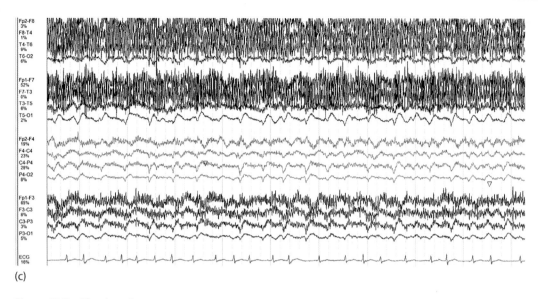

(c)

Figure 16.2   (Continued)

In cases of ED frequency ≤2.5 Hz or rhythmic delta/theta activity >0.5 Hz, "possible NCSE" can be diagnosed when:

1. There is no spatiotemporal evolution, but fluctuations are seen or,
2. There is EEG improvement without clinical improvement following IV antiseizure medication administration.

Patients with known encephalopathy

Patients with a background history of epileptic encephalopathy need to satisfy one of the following criteria in addition to the usual criteria of NCSE mentioned previously.

1. Increased activity (in amplitude or frequency) compared with the baseline.
2. Clinical and EEG improvement with IV antiseizure medications.

ELECTROGRAPHIC VERSUS ELECTROCLINICAL STATUS EPILEPTICUS

Finally, it is important to understand the difference between electrographic and electroclinical status epilepticus as defined by the American Clinical Neurophysiology Society.[8] Electrographic SE, based on the EEG, is not associated with any clinical semiology and is defined as an electrographic seizure continuing for ≥10 minutes or total seizure activity accounting for ≥20% of a 60-minute EEG recording. Possible electrographic SE overlaps with ictal-interictal continuum (IIC) patterns of periodic discharges, spike/sharp wave discharges, and rhythmic delta activity (except generalized rhythmic delta activity). Electroclinical seizures are characterized by ictal EEG patterns time-locked with clinical correlates. When an electroclinical seizure continues for ≥10 minutes or total seizure activity within a 60-minute EEG accounts for ≥20% of the recording, electroclinical SE is diagnosed. An exception to the rule is bilateral tonic-clonic seizure activity which must continue for ≥5 minutes only to satisfy the criteria for electroclinical SE. When a rhythmic or periodic pattern of IIC continues for ≥10 minutes or occupies ≥20% of the 60-minute EEG recording, possible electroclinical SE can be diagnosed if the EEG improves, without associated clinical improvement, with the administration of a parenteral antiseizure medication. If both EEG and clinical improvement is achieved with parenteral antiseizure medication, definite electroclinical SE is diagnosed.[8]

References

1. Trinka, E, Cock, H, Hesdorffer, D, Rossetti, AO, Scheffer, IE, Shinnar, S, et al. A definition and classification of status epilepticus–Report of the ILAE Task Force on Classification of Status Epilepticus. Epilepsia 2015;56:1515–1523.

2. Manfredonia, F, Saturno, E, Lawley, A, Gasverde, S, Cavanna, AE. Prevalence and clinical correlates of non-convulsive status epilepticus in elderly patients with acute confusional state: A systematic literature review. J Neurol Sci 2020;410:116674.

3. Sutter, R, Ruegg, S, Kaplan, PW. Epidemiology, diagnosis, and management of nonconvulsive status epilepticus: Opening Pandora's box. Neurol Clin Pract 2012;2:275–286.

4. Mutis, JA, Rodríguez, JH, Nava-Mesa, MO. Rapidly progressive cognitive impairment with neuropsychiatric symptoms as the initial manifestation of status epilepticus. Epilepsy Behav Case Rep 2017; 7:20–23.

5. Profitlich, T, Hoppe, C, Reuber, M, Helmstaedter, C, Bauer, J. Ictal neuropsychological findings in focal nonconvulsive status epilepticus. Epilepsy Behav 2008;12:269–275.

6. Covanis, A. Panayiotopoulos syndrome: A benign childhood autonomic epilepsy frequently imitating encephalitis, syncope, migraine, sleep disorder, or gastroenteritis. Pediatrics 2006;118:e1237–1243.

7. Leitinger, M, Beniczky, S, Rohracher, A, Gardella, E, Kalss, G, Qerama, E, et al. Salzburg Consensus Criteria for Non-Convulsive Status Epilepticus–approach to clinical application. Epilepsy Behav 2015; 49:158–163.

8. Hirsch, LJ, Fong, MWK, Leitinger, M, et al. American Clinical Neurophysiology Society's standardized critical care EEG terminology: 2021 Version. J Clin Neurophysiol 2021;38(1):1–29.

CHAPTER 17

EEG in encephalopathy and coma

ETIOPATHOGENESIS

Encephalopathy generally refers to an altered mental state manifesting with impaired consciousness and cognition to varying degrees, indicating a diffuse disturbance in brain function.[1] In terms of severity, encephalopathy represents a spectrum ranging from subtle changes in cognition to deep coma. It can be acute, subacute, or chronic. Clinically, it is not uncommon to witness a waxing and waning course in some cases.

The electroencephalogram (EEG) changes in encephalopathy reflect the location, extent, and severity of the involvement of anatomical structures in the pathological process. As described in Chapter 4, cortical dysfunction leads to posterior background slowing and decreased EEG amplitude. Rhythmic or arrhythmic delta slowing and triphasic waves represent the dysfunction of the subcortical white matter. The brainstem involvement results in generalized slowing as well as abnormal arousal patterns and spindle activity.[2]

The etiologies of encephalopathy are variable and difficult to differentiate based on the EEG. The common etiologies encountered in different settings include:

1. Toxic: Alcohol, illicit drugs, other medications (particularly polypharmacy), chemicals, drug, and alcohol withdrawal.

2. Metabolic: Organ failure (liver, kidney, lung), electrolyte disturbances, endocrine abnormalities.

3. Hypoxia.

4. Infections: Central nervous system or systemic including sepsis.

5. Cerebrovascular disease: Ischemic or hemorrhagic.

6. Inflammatory and autoimmune: Encephalitis, vasculitis.

7. Structural: Brain tumor, hydrocephalus.

8. Post-traumatic: Acute or chronic.

9. Postictal state.

10. Neurodegenerative illnesses: Dementia, Creutzfeldt-Jakob disease.

EEG PATTERNS OF ENCEPHALOPATHY

Slowing of the posterior dominant rhythm

The slowing of the posterior dominant rhythm (PDR) is an early sign of mild encephalopathy. There may be intrusions of theta slowing into the alpha rhythm that are still reactive. As encephalopathy progresses, alpha rhythms are completely replaced by slow activity.

DOI: 10.1201/9781003353713-21

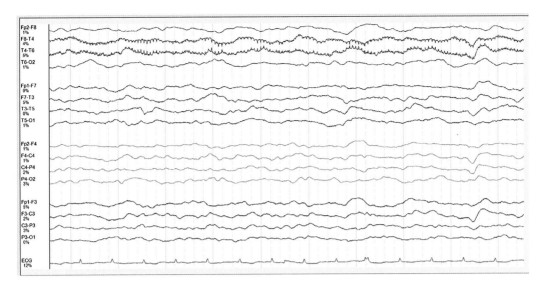

Figure 17.1 Generalized theta and delta slowing.

Generalized theta slowing

With advancing encephalopathy, the recording predominantly consists of generalized theta slowing. Less than 20% of the EEG contains alpha and delta activity during wakefulness.[3] The reactive PDR disappears with deeper stages of encephalopathy.

Generalized theta-delta slowing

During this stage, the background consists of predominantly generalized theta admixed with delta activity with <20% of the EEG showing alpha intrusions (Figure 17.1).[3] Though this pattern is not specific to any particular etiology, one study found theta-delta patterns to be significantly associated with intracranial hemorrhages and unfavorable outcomes.[3]

Generalized delta slowing

As encephalopathy deepens, >80% of the recording consists of generalized delta activity.[3] Delta slowing can be arrhythmic or rhythmic.

Frontal intermittent delta activity (FIRDA) is now included under the umbrella of generalized rhythmic delta activity (GRDA) in the American Clinical Neurophysiology Society (ACNS) terminology as "GRDA with frontal predominance."[4] FIRDA is characterized by bi-frontally dominant rhythmic delta waves of ≤4 Hz with uniform morphology and duration.[4] Furthermore, to satisfy the criterion of "rhythmic," the delta activity should persist for at least six cycles (e.g., 3 Hz delta should last 2 seconds).[4] However, FIRDA is a non-specific pattern found in many conditions, including toxic and metabolic encephalopathies, hypoxic encephalopathy, epileptic encephalopathy, neurodegenerative diseases, systemic and CNS infections, structural brain lesions (tumors, stroke, hemorrhage, leukoencephalopathy), and during hyperventilation in healthy individuals.[5,6]

Triphasic waves

First described in patients with hepatic encephalopathy, triphasic waves can be seen in a plethora of conditions. In ACNS terminology, triphasic waves are defined as complexes with (1) two or three phases, (2) the duration of each phase is longer than the preceding phase, and (3) the maximum amplitude is recorded by the positive phase.[4] When there are three phases, the sequence should be negative-positive-negative, whereas it is positive-negative in cases with only two phases.[4] Anterior-posterior or posterior-anterior time lag is often observed. The lag is defined as >100 ms

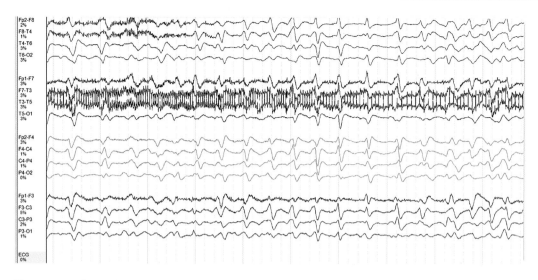

Figure 17.2   Generalized periodic triphasic waves. This EEG was recorded from an encephalopathic patient with renal failure. Note the triphasic waves with anterior-posterior lag.

time difference between the most anterior and most posterior EEG derivations in both the longitudinal bipolar and referential montages (Figure 17.2).[4] The distribution of triphasic waves can vary from focal, lateralized, bilateral independent, and multifocal to generalized. The occurrence of triphasic waves can be periodic or non-periodic. Triphasic waves are included under the umbrella of "periodic discharges" in ACNS terminology.[4]

The best-known association of triphasic waves is encephalopathy, both acute and chronic, where the distribution of triphasic waves is typically generalized. Creutzfeldt-Jakob disease is a chronic condition well-known to be associated with periodic triphasic waves. A study on triphasic waves in acute encephalopathy found white matter lesions in 60% and brain atrophy in 59% of patients.[7] In this study, infections and renal, hepatic, as well as respiratory failure were the most frequently encountered etiologies.[7] Ninety-six percent had generalized triphasic waves with 73% showing fronto-central maxima. Most patients demonstrated both the anterior-posterior and posterior-anterior time lag. In the vast majority, the frequency of triphasic waves was either increased or decreased with external noxious stimuli with only 16% showing no change. The lack of background EEG reactivity was found to be a significant predictor of death.[7]

It is important to emphasize that triphasic waves are not specific for encephalopathy. It has been reported in association with non-convulsive status epilepticus (NCSE).[8] It is particularly challenging to differentiate encephalopathy from NCSE when triphasic waves occur in the form of generalized periodic discharges (GPD). Several studies have attempted to identify morphological features of triphasic waves in GPD to differentiate those associated with seizures from encephalopathy. Shorter duration of the waveform, sharp morphology, lower amplitude of phase II with dominant phase I, fronto-polar maxima (as opposed to fronto-central maxima), higher frequency (>1 Hz), the lack of anterior-posterior lag, and the lack of frequency change with stimulation are considered to be features of triphasic waves associated with a seizure risk.[9] However, none of these features can make a definitive distinction. To confirm or refute the diagnosis of NCSE, the diagnostic criteria (discussed in Chapter 16) should be applied. If the GPD conforms to the entity of ictal-interictal continuum, the 2HELPS2B tool (discussed in Chapter 15) can be applied to estimate the associated seizure risk.

Furthermore, triphasic waves have been described in association with structural brain abnormalities without encephalopathy.[10] Focal triphasic waves can be a rare interictal abnormality in epilepsy.[11]

Cyclic alternating pattern of encephalopathy

The cyclic alternating pattern seen in encephalopathy and coma (CAPE) should not be mistaken for the cyclic alternating pattern (CAP) in sleep. CAPE is characterized by spontaneously alternating two background patterns in a regular manner continuing for six or more cycles. Each background pattern should last ≥10 seconds. A cycle is defined as the total duration of the two sequential background patterns. This pattern is different from burst suppression. CAPE can be seen in encephalopathy of any etiology. The prognostic significance of CAPE has not been well studied and a small case series reported a good prognosis with ten out of 11 surviving the coma and five patients achieving a good functional recovery.[12]

EEG PATTERNS OF COMA

Coma refers to a state of prolonged unconsciousness, characterized by the absence of arousal and awareness as a result of dysfunction of the arousal system involving the reticular activating system, thalamic connections, and cerebral cortex. Typically, eyes remain closed, the sleep-wake cycle is abnormal, and the person is non-rousable in coma. The structural causes of coma include damage to bilateral cerebral hemispheres and ascending reticular activating system (midbrain, pons, bilateral thalami/hypothalamic). Raised intracranial pressure causes coma by affecting the ascending reticular activating system. Toxic, metabolic, and hypoxic encephalopathies result in coma as a result of depression and dysfunction of the cerebral cortex (bilateral) and reticular activating system.[13] The Glasgow Coma Scale is a useful tool to monitor the progress of coma.

EEG is invaluable in the diagnosis, assessment of severity, and prognostication of coma. Several EEG patterns have been described in comatose patients. Slower frequencies and lower waveform amplitudes are associated with poor prognosis.[14] However, across many studies, the best prognostic marker has been found to be the EEG reactivity to external stimuli. EEG reactivity to external noise and sternal rubbing appears to be the best prognostic indicators of good outcomes following hypoxic brain injury due to cardiac arrest.[15]

Alpha coma

The alpha coma pattern is characterized by monomorphic generalized alpha-range activity (8–13 Hz) with bifrontal or posterior maxima (Figure 17.3). There is no spontaneous variability and minimum or no reactivity. This pattern is seen in hypoxic, toxic, and metabolic encephalopathies as well as brainstem (pons/medulla) lesions. The prognosis usually depends on the etiology with hypoxic encephalopathy carrying a worse prognosis than alpha coma due to drug overdose.

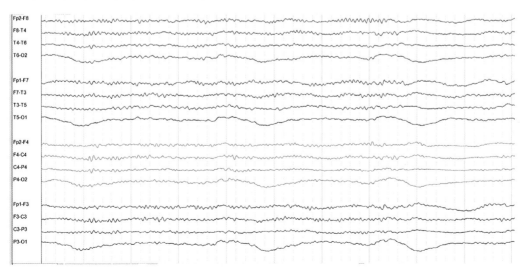

Figure 17.3 Alpha coma pattern.

Beta coma

The beta coma pattern is characterized by generalized 12–16 Hz activity, often with a bifrontal emphasis. Though beta is the predominant rhythm, other frequencies may be seen intermittently admixed in the background. Reactivity to external stimuli varies depending on the severity of coma with the complete absence of reactivity noted in deep coma. The most common etiology of a beta coma is drug intoxication.

Theta coma

In theta coma, the predominant rhythm is generalized rhythmic theta activity usually with frontal maxima.[16] As in alpha and beta comas, reactivity to stimuli is determined by the severity of coma. This pattern can be seen in hypoxic encephalopathies.

Delta coma

Delta coma is characterized by generalized delta activity, which can be polymorphic or rhythmic with a frontal emphasis (Figure 17.4).[17] Two patterns based on the amplitude have been described: low-voltage (<50 microvolts) and medium to high-voltage (≥50 microvolts) coma. The reactivity disappears as the coma deepens. The etiology varies from metabolic encephalopathy, raised intracranial pressure, infections, trauma, and hypoxic-ischemic encephalopathy.

Spindle coma

In spindle coma, bilateral symmetric and synchronous bursts of 11–14 Hz spindle activity emerge paroxysmally on a slow background.[18] This pattern has been described in encephalopathies of varying etiologies and structural abnormalities in the brain stem. The prognosis in spindle coma usually depends on the underlying etiology.

Burst suppression

The burst suppression pattern represents a severe form of encephalopathy commonly seen in the setting of hypoxic encephalopathy, but by no means specific to any particular etiology (Figure 17.5). Therapeutic burst suppression with anesthetic agents is an option to treat refractory status epilepticus. This pattern is characterized by alternating "bursts" of EEG waveforms and periods of "EEG suppression." According to the ACNS terminology, to qualify for burst suppression, 50–99% of the EEG record should contain suppression. On average, bursts should last ≥0.5 and ≤30 seconds with four or more phases.[4] If these criteria are not fulfilled, the waveform is considered a "discharge" rather than a "burst" and the pattern will be labeled "periodic discharges." Bursts may consist of any

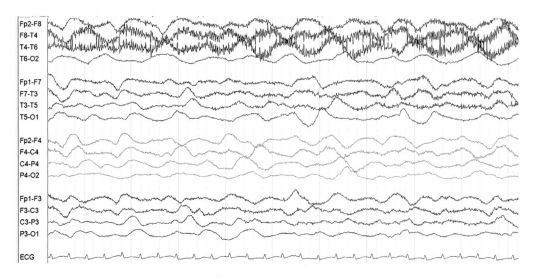

Figure 17.4   Delta coma pattern. This EEG was recorded from a patient in coma caused by a drug overdose.

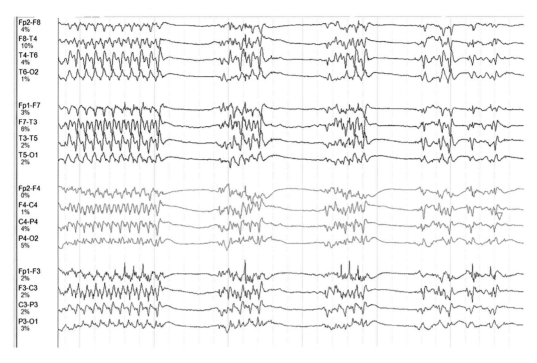

Figure 17.5   The burst suppression pattern in hypoxic-ischemic encephalopathy due to cardiac arrest.

EEG waveform, including epileptiform discharges, of ≥10 microvolts. Highly epileptiform bursts are defined as the presence of two or more epileptiform discharges with an average frequency of ≥1 Hz within a burst in >50% of the bursts.[4] The suppression is defined as periods of EEG voltage <10 microvolts.[4] When describing the burst suppression pattern, burst duration, burst components, inter-burst interval, and the percentage of the EEG record showing suppression should be specified.

Generalized suppression

When the EEG record consists of activity with amplitude <10 microvolts, generalized suppression is diagnosed (Figure 17.6). Attenuation is defined as EEG activity of ≥10 microvolts, but <50% of the background voltage.[4] If >99% of the EEG record shows suppression/attenuation, it is labeled

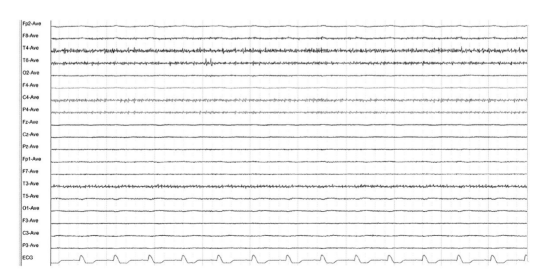

Figure 17.6   Generalized EEG suppression in hypoxic-ischemic encephalopathy due to cardiac arrest.

as continuous suppression/attenuation, whereas 10–49% period is identified as discontinuous.[4] Continuous generalized suppression represents a very severe stage of coma.

Electrocerebral inactivity

Electrocerebral inactivity (ECI) or isoelectric EEG is the irreversible end-stage of coma with EEG showing a "flatline" with the peak-to-peak voltage <2 microvolts. However, to diagnose ECI and brain death, the EEG should be recorded in accordance with strict guidelines.[19] In summary, the EEG recording must ensure adequate scalp electrode coverage with an interelectrode distance of ≤10 cm, interelectrode impedance 100–10,000 ohms, recording sensitivity up to 2 microvolts/mm, and proper filter setting (high-frequency filter ≥30 Hz and low-frequency filter ≤1 Hz).[19]

GRADING OF EEG PATTERNS IN ENCEPHALOPATHY AND COMA

There is no universally accepted grading scale for encephalopathy and coma. Synek proposed five grades in 1988.[16]

1. Predominant alpha activity with intermittent and reactive theta slowing.

2. Predominant theta activity admixed with occasional alpha and delta.

3. Predominant delta activity, arrhythmic or rhythmic (including FIRDA), and small-amplitude.

4. Burst suppression, alpha coma, and theta coma.

5. Electrocerebral inactivity.

Small-amplitude grade 3, grade 4, and grade 5 patterns are considered "malignant" patterns, indicating poor prognosis.[16]

HYPOXIC-ISCHEMIC ENCEPHALOPATHY

Hypoxic-ischemic encephalopathy (HIE) is a major cause of mortality among patients admitted to the intensive care unit following a cardiac arrest. The withdrawal of life-sustaining treatment is usually guided by neuroprognostication. Multimodal prognostication based on clinical assessment, electrophysiology (EEG, somatosensory evoked potential), neuroimaging, and biomarkers (neuron-specific enolase) is recommended in the guidelines.[20] EEG plays an important role in prognostication. The EEG changes in HIE range from background slowing to electrocerebral inactivity, as in other encephalopathies. However, specific EEG patterns in HIE useful in neuroprognostication merit discussion here.

Some authors have defined "highly malignant" and "malignant" EEG patterns in HIE. Highly malignant patterns are background suppression with or without periodic discharges and burst suppression. Malignant EEG patterns include (a) abundant periodic or rhythmic discharges, (b) electrographic seizures or status epilepticus, (c) low-voltage (<20 microvolts) background, (d) discontinuous background where >10% of the recording consists of background suppression, (e) reversal of anterior-posterior gradient or alpha coma pattern, and (f) loss of background reactivity.[21] In one study, highly malignant EEG patterns predicted poor neurological outcomes with 98% specificity and 31% sensitivity. Malignant rhythmic, periodic, or seizure patterns had higher specificity (96%) than malignant background alterations (80%) for poor outcomes.[22]

In a meta-analysis of pooled data, burst suppression (specificity 98%, sensitivity 31%), electrocerebral inactivity (specificity 98.5%, sensitivity 13.5%), electrographic status epilepticus (specificity 98%, sensitivity 22%), and generalized periodic discharges (specificity 92%, sensitivity 38%) captured on the EEG performed within 24 hours of admission or cardiac arrest predicted death and disability in HIE.[23]

Only a few studies have evaluated EEG-derived quantitative indices in this setting. One study defined the background continuity index (BCI) as the proportion of EEG record without background suppression, whereas the burst suppression amplitude ratio (BSAR) was defined as the ratio between the standard deviations of signal amplitudes outside and within suppression periods.[24] Higher BCI and lower BSAR were in favor of a good outcome. A model combining BCI and BSAR predicted a good outcome at 24 hours with 90% specificity and 57% sensitivity.[24] Another study proposed a score, labeled as the NEC2RAS score, based on six EEG parameters: EEG at 12–36 hours (1) no epileptiform abnormalities, (2) continuity of background ≥50%, (3) reactivity; EEG at 36–72 hrs (4) reactivity, (5) normal background amplitude, and (6) stimulus-induced rhythmic, periodic, or ictal discharges (SIRPIDs). Each EEG feature was assigned one point. Scores of 2 or higher predicted recovery of consciousness outside the vegetative state with 100% sensitivity and 70% specificity.[25]

Early myoclonus is considered a poor prognostic sign and one study reported 97% specificity in predicting death.[26] However, favorable outcomes among patients with myoclonus have been reported and good outcomes were significantly less frequent when myoclonus was accompanied by epileptiform abnormalities on the EEG.[27] Myoclonus can be cortical or subcortical in origin. It is important to differentiate acute post-anoxic myoclonus from Lance-Adams syndrome, which has a more favorable prognosis. Generalized tonic-clonic, myoclonic, non-convulsive, and electrographic seizures have been reported among patients with HIE. Additionally, EEG patterns of the ictal-interictal continuum are well recognized in this population. In a randomized prospective study, suppression of rhythmic and periodic discharges with antiseizure medications did not significantly change the outcome at three months.[28] However, this study included both status epilepticus and non-ictal rhythmic and periodic patterns. Though status epilepticus is considered a poor prognostic factor, it should be emphasized that favorable outcomes with the treatment of status epilepticus, particularly non-convulsive status epilepticus, have been reported.

The European Resuscitation Council and the European Society of Intensive Care Medicine have published guidelines on prognostication following cardiac arrest and resuscitation.[29] Six prognostic markers have been defined: (1) absence of corneal and pupillary reflexes at ≥72 hours, (2) absence of N20 in somatosensory evoked potentials bilaterally at ≥24 hours, (3) neuron specific enolase >60 µg/L at 48–72 hours, (4) EEG burst suppression or background suppression at >24 hours, (5) status myoclonus at ≤72 hours, and (6) diffuse anoxic injury on neuroimaging. The presence of two or more of those markers predicts a poor outcome.[29]

References

1. Markand, ON. Electroencephalography in diffuse encephalopathies. J Clin Neurophysiol 1984;1:357–407.

2. Kaplan, PW, Rossetti, AO. EEG patterns and imaging correlations in Encephalopathy: Encephalopathy part II. J Clin Neurophysiol 2011;28:233–251.

3. Sutter, R, Stevens, RD, Kaplan, PW. Clinical and imaging correlates of EEG patterns in hospitalized patients with encephalopathy. J Neurol 2013;260:1087–1098.

4. Hirsch, LJ, Fong, MWK, Leitinger, M, et al. American Clinical Neurophysiology Society's standardized critical care EEG Terminology: 2021 Version. J Clin Neurophysiol 2021;38(1):1–29.

5. Accolla, EA, Kaplan, PW, Maeder-Ingvar, M, Jukopila, S, Rossetti, AO. Clinical correlates of frontal intermittent rhythmic delta activity (FIRDA). Clin Neurophysiol 2011;122:27–31.

6. Kim, KT, Roh, Y-N, Cho, NH, Jeon, JC. Clinical correlates of frontal intermittent rhythmic delta activity without structural brain lesion. Clin EEG Neurosci 2021;52:69–73.

7. Sutter, R, Stevens, RD, Kaplan, PW. Significance of triphasic waves in patients with acute encephalopathy: A nine-year cohort study. Clin Neurophysiol 2013;124:1952–1958.

8. Kaya, D, Bingol, CA. Significance of atypical triphasic waves for diagnosing nonconvulsive status epilepticus. Epilepsy Behav 2007;11:567–577.

9. Hartshorn, JA, Foreman, B. Generalized periodic discharges with triphasic morphology. J Neurocrit Care 2019;12:1–8.

10. Aguglia, U, Gambardella, A, Oliveri, RL, Lavano, A, Quattrone, A. Nonmetabolic causes of triphasic waves: A reappraisal. Clin Electroencephalogr 1990;21:120–125.

11. Janati AB, ALGhasab NS, Aldaife MY, et al. Atypical interictal epileptiform discharges in electroencephalography. J Epilepsy Res 2018;8:55–60.

12. Kassab, MY, Farooq, MU, Diaz-Arrastia, R, Van Ness, PC. The clinical significance of EEG cyclic alternating pattern during coma. J Clin Neurophysiol 2007;24:425–428.

13. Bateman, DE. Neurological assessment of coma. J Neurol Neurosurg Psychiatry 2001;71:i13–i17.

14. Bagnato, S, Boccagni, C, Sant'Angelo, A, Prestandrea, C, Mazzilli, R, Galardi, G. EEG predictors of outcome in patients with disorders of consciousness admitted for intensive rehabilitation. Clin Neurophysiol 2015;126:959–966.

15. Admiraal, MM, Horn, J, Hofmeijer, J, et al. EEG reactivity testing for prediction of good outcome in patients after cardiac arrest. Neurology 2020;95:e653–e661.

16. Synek, VM. Prognostically important EEG coma patterns in diffuse anoxic and traumatic encephalopathies in adults. J Clin Neurophysiol 1988;5:161–174.

17. Sutter, R, Kaplan, PW. Clinical and electroencephalographic correlates of acute encephalopathy. J Clin Neurophysiol 2013;30:443–453.

18. Kaplan, PW. The EEG in metabolic encephalopathy and coma. J Clin Neurophysiol 2004;21:307–318.

19. Stecker, MM, Sabau, D, Sullivan, L, et al. American Clinical Neurophysiology Society Guideline 6: Minimum technical standards for EEG recording in suspected cerebral death. J Clin Neurophysiol 2016;33:324–327.

20. Nolan, JP, Soar, J, Cariou, A, et al. European Resuscitation Council and European Society of Intensive Care Medicine 2015 guidelines for post-resuscitation care. Intensive Care Med 2015;41:2039–2056.

21. Westhall, E, Rosén, I, Rossetti, AO, et al. Electroencephalography (EEG) for neurological prognostication after cardiac arrest and targeted temperature management; Rationale and study design. BMC Neurology 2014;14:159.

22. Backman, S, Cronberg, T, Friberg, H, et al. Highly malignant routine EEG predicts poor prognosis after cardiac arrest in the target temperature management trial. Resuscitation 2018;131:24–28.

23. Perera, K, Khan, S, Singh, S, et al. EEG patterns and outcomes after hypoxic brain injury: A systematic review and meta-analysis. Neurocrit Care 2022;36:292–301.

24. Ruijter, BJ, Hofmeijer, J, Tjepkema-Cloostermans, MC, van Putten, MJAM. The prognostic value of discontinuous EEG patterns in postanoxic coma. Clin Neurophysiol 2018;129:1534–1543.

25. Barbella, G, Lee, JW, Alvarez, V, et al. Prediction of regaining consciousness despite an early epileptiform EEG after cardiac arrest. Neurology 2020;94:e1675–e1683.

26. Rossetti, AO, Oddo, M, Logroscino, G, Kaplan, PW. Prognostication after cardiac arrest and hypothermia: A prospective study. Ann Neurol 2010;67:301–307.

27. Seder, DB, Sunde, K, Rubertsson, S, et al. Neurologic outcomes and postresuscitation care of patients with myoclonus following cardiac arrest. Crit Care Med 2015;43:965–972.

28. Ruijter, BJ, Keijzer, HM, Tjepkema-Cloostermans, MC, et al. Treating rhythmic and periodic EEG patterns in comatose survivors of cardiac arrest. N Engl J Med 2022;386:724–734.

29. Nolan, JP, Sandroni, C, Böttiger, BW, et al. European Resuscitation Council and European Society of Intensive Care Medicine Guidelines 2021: Post-resuscitation care. Intensive Care Med 2021;47:369–421.

CHAPTER 18

A systematic approach to the critical care EEG

INTRODUCTION AND KEY STEPS

There are multiple challenges in reading critical care electroencephalograms (EEGs). First, the nature of the environment and the patient population in the ICU setting make the EEG susceptible to a multitude of artifacts. Second, patients are likely to be on multiple medications, including sedatives, rendering the interpretation of EEG changes very difficult. Third, the EEG patterns are complex and distinctively different from routine outpatient EEGs. Finally, critical management decisions may depend on the EEG and the electroencephalographer has a responsibility to provide an accurate, precise, and timely report. Reading critical care EEGs needs additional training and a skillset beyond routine EEG reporting.

It is also important to highlight that not all EEGs recorded in the ICU are abnormal. For example, patients with psychogenic non-epileptic seizures may be admitted to the ICU with suspected status epilepticus and those EEGs are likely to be normal except for movement and muscle artifacts.

Given the complexity of the EEG, it is useful to adopt a systematic approach to cover all aspects of a critical care EEG. The following scheme highlights a rational step-by-step approach with the hope of providing a reliable and practical framework to beginners for reading critical care EEGs.

1. Find out the background medical information

Background history is critical in interpreting the EEG in the ICU. There are several important questions to ask before looking at the EEG: what is the suspected diagnosis? What is the indication for EEG: diagnosis or prognostication? What is the level of consciousness of the patient? What medications is the patient on? Is the patient on any sedation or anesthetic agents and was it ceased before the EEG recording? If ceased, how long before the EEG recording commenced? The EEG reader should study this information carefully before going through the EEG record. Burst suppression in a patient on propofol is not interpreted the same way as burst suppression due to hypoxic encephalopathy. If the question is about prognostication after hypoxic brain injury, it is important to know when the event occurred, and the EEG should be recorded off sedation. On the other hand, if the question is about the adequacy of therapeutic burst suppression in status epilepticus, the EEG should be recorded while the usual anesthetic infusion is running, and the reader should note the agent as well as the dosage at the time of EEG.

2. Look for a posterior dominant rhythm

The first step in reading the critical care EEG is to look for a posterior dominant background rhythm. If present, it indicates retained alertness of the subject and the EEG is likely to be uncomplicated.

DOI: 10.1201/9781003353713-22

3. Look for interictal epileptiform discharges

As you go through each epoch, carefully look for EEG abnormalities. Interictal epileptiform discharges are easy to detect. Those can be generalized, focal, multifocal, or lateralized. Details of interictal epileptiform discharges have been discussed in Chapter 9.

4. Look for ictal patterns

One of the key diagnostic considerations of critical care EEG is electrographic ictal rhythms. Look for evolving ictal patterns as detailed in Chapters 9 and 16. Review the video for semiology, study the annotations by the technologist, and correlate with the ictal rhythm.

5. Look for patterns of the ictal-interictal continuum

Patterns of IIC represent a spectrum of electrographic changes rather than a unifying diagnosis as detailed in Chapter 15. The spectrum of IIC includes periodic discharges (lateralized, bilateral independent, generalized), rhythmic delta activity (lateralized, generalized), brief potentially ictal rhythmic discharges (B[I]RDs), and stimulus-induced rhythmic, periodic, or ictal discharges (SIRPIDs). These patterns should be carefully looked for and described in detail across multiple domains.

- Topography
- Prevalence
- Frequency
- Morphology (triphasic-look for A-P or P-A lag)
- Amplitude (<20 microvolts = very low, 20–49 microvolts = low, 50–149 microvolts = medium, and ≥150 microvolts = high)
- Polarity
- Stimulus induced/terminated or not
- Fluctuating versus evolving
- Plus features

Please read Chapter 15 for more information.

6. Look for slowing

Keep looking for non-epileptiform EEG abnormalities in each epoch. Slowing is one such abnormality. Describe the characteristic of slowing.

- The distribution: Posterior background, focal, multifocal, regional, hemispheric, generalized.
- Amplitude.
- Frequency: Theta, delta.
- Persistence of slowing: Intermittent versus continuous.
- Rhythmicity (rhythmic versus arrhythmic): Slow waves of the same duration (frequency) occurring in runs are considered rhythmic.
- Regularity (regular versus irregular): Slow waves of the same morphology occurring in runs are considered regular (monomorphic). When the morphology is variable, it is called irregular (polymorphic).
- Reactivity: Variability of slowing with stimuli or the state of vigilance is referred to as reactivity.

7. Look for attenuation in activity

Attenuation is another important non-epileptiform abnormality. Attenuation can be generalized or focal. See Chapter 13 for details.

8. Look for enhanced activity

As described in Chapter 13, increased activity can be focal or generalized. Focally increased activity due to breach rhythm is particularly relevant in the ICU setting where patients with previous neurosurgery are admitted due to reduced conscious state.

9. Look for specific patterns of encephalopathy and coma

Patterns of encephalopathy and coma are described in detail in Chapter 17. This includes different degrees of slowing, triphasic waves, cyclic alternating pattern, alpha coma, beta coma, theta coma, delta coma, spindle coma, burst suppression, and generalized suppression.

10. Look for signs of reactivity

Reactivity is an important prognostic marker of the critical care EEG and is defined as reproducible changes in EEG amplitude or frequency with stimulation. First and foremost, reactivity may be visible in the ICU with routine stimulations, such as nursing care, suction of secretions, and cannulation. The electroencephalographer should carefully look for EEG changes with such stimulation. More importantly, the technologist should carefully test for reactivity with a standard protocol. One such protocol describes reactivity testing in four domains: auditory (clapping and calling out name), tactile (stimulation of the nasal septum with a cotton swab), visual (passive eye opening), and pain (sternal pressure). Each stimulus should be applied for 5 seconds and repeated at 30-second intervals three times in a row. When one or more (out of five) stimuli produce a clear change in EEG amplitude or frequency at least twice (of the three trains of stimulations), the presence of EEG reactivity is confirmed.[1,2] Other studies have included intermittent photic stimulation also as a testing method, but reactivity to photic stimulation does not appear to be a predictor of favorable outcomes.[3]

11. Ensure reading with more than one montage

It is a mistake to read any EEG using a single montage. This is particularly relevant to critical care EEGs. The longitudinal bipolar montage is a great option for screening the EEG, particularly when there are rhythmic patterns of high amplitude. However, a referential montage should be used to study the morphology, amplitude, and voltage fields. This is particularly helpful in visualizing evolving ictal patterns. The transverse bipolar montage is valuable in studying the details of abnormalities in the central region and midline.

12. Do not be afraid to change the EEG settings, but know the limitations

Changing the digital EEG settings such as filters, sensitivity, and timebase can greatly enhance the yield. For example, compressing the timebase can increase the visibility of periodic patterns. However, these manipulations are fraught with potential dangers and the reader should approach them rationally.[4]

13. Beware of blind spots

In any EEG epoch, there are four potential blind spots where abnormalities can be easily overlooked: (1) beginning of the epoch, (2) end of the epoch, (3) top margin, and (4) bottom of the page (Figure 18.1). The top margin of the epoch can be particularly tricky – with eye movements and undulations, the EEG channel intermittently becomes not visible. End-of-the-chain abnormalities can be easily missed if multiple montages are not used. The same applies to the bottom of the epoch and one must pay particular attention to the ECG rhythm strip.

14. Study the video carefully and correlate behavioral events with the EEG

Patients in the ICU may exhibit many behaviors other than epileptic seizures. The spectrum includes psychogenic non-epileptic seizures, stereotypic movements seen in autoimmune encephalitis, roving eye movements of encephalopathy, movement disorders, and myoclonic jerks.

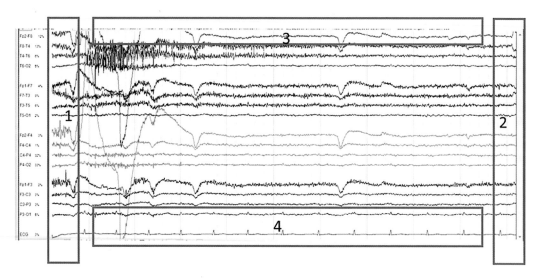

Figure 18.1   The four "blind spots" in an EEG epoch.

One study has found that 78% of behavioral changes and movements, including tremor-like movements, slow semi-purposeful movements, multifocal myoclonus, abnormal eye movements, and repetitive behaviors, such as head banging, clonus, and facial twitching, are not seizure-related movements.[5] Movements mimicking seizures have been well reported with propofol therapy.[6] Therefore, the electroencephalographer must study and correlate these phenomena very carefully.

15. Be mindful of misinterpretation of artifacts

The ICU environment is not very friendly for EEG recording and artifacts are not uncommon. The reader must be very careful not to misinterpret artifacts. It is always helpful to look at the video and the annotations made by the technologist. More details on this topic can be found in Chapter 7.

16. Take time and review again

Critical care EEGs are complex and cannot be read in a rush. The reader should allocate sufficient time to go through the EEG. Whenever there is a doubt, such regions must be reviewed more than once. It is also helpful to discuss with a colleague when a complex EEG is encountered.

17. Classify the abnormality

Having carefully reviewed the EEG, the electroencephalographer must classify the EEG in preparation to generate the report. The EEG can be normal or abnormal. It is also useful to grade the degree of abnormality objectively.

18. Summarize the findings

It is very useful to summarize the abnormalities in a logical manner.

- Epileptiform abnormalities:
  - Interictal
  - Ictal
  - Ictal-interictal continuum
- Non-epileptiform abnormalities:
  - Slowing
  - Attenuation
  - Enhancement
  - Patterns of encephalopathy and coma

19. Interpret the findings and provide clinical correlation

This is a critical component of the EEG report. Bear in mind that there may be clinicians who only read this section to get a quick idea about what is wrong with the patient. Hence, the interpretation must be succinct and easily understood. Main interpretations may include the following:

- Encephalopathy/coma
- Structural abnormality or dysfunction
- Interictal
  - Focal or generalized epileptogenicity
- Ictal
  - Isolated seizure
  - Seizure clusters
  - Status epilepticus
- Ictal-interictal continuum
  - Provide risk prediction using 2HELPS2B score[7]

The clinical interpretation of the EEG findings is an integral part of the EEG reporting. It should explicitly express the clinical relevance of the findings in a language understood by the referring clinician. Ambiguous terminology should be avoided. EEG is a test, not a consult, hence, suggestions on patient management should be avoided. However, it may be appropriate to suggest further testing such as video-EEG monitoring, ECG monitoring, and repeating the EEG, depending on the findings.

20. Generate the report

Generating the report is the final step in the process. Do not hesitate to review the EEG again and again, whenever there is any doubt, before finalizing the report. The American Clinical Neurophysiology Society has published guidelines on EEG reporting.[8] Essential components of an EEG report are described in Chapter 4.

References

1. Admiraal, MM, Horn, J, Hofmeijer, J, Hoedemaekers, CWE, van Kaam, CR, Keijzer, HM, et al. EEG reactivity testing for prediction of good outcome in patients after cardiac arrest. Neurology 2020; 95:e653–e661.

2. Admiraal, MM, van Rootselaar, AF, Hofmeijer, J, Hoedemaekers, CWE, van Kaam, CR, Keijzer, HM, et al. Electroencephalographic reactivity as predictor of neurological outcome in postanoxic coma: A multicenter prospective cohort study. Ann Neurol 2019;86:17–27.

3. Estraneo, A, Fiorenza, S, Magliacano, A, Formisano, R, Mattia, D, Grippo, A, et al. Multicenter prospective study on predictors of short-term outcome in disorders of consciousness. Neurology 2020;95:e1488–e1499.

4. Seneviratne, U. Rational manipulation of digital EEG: Pearls and pitfalls. J Clin Neurophysiol 2014; 31:507–516.

5. Benbadis, SR, Chen, S, Melo, M. What's shaking in the ICU? The differential diagnosis of seizures in the intensive care setting. Epilepsia 2010;51:2338–2340.

6. Walder, B, Tramèr, MR, Seeck, M. Seizure-like phenomena and propofol: A systematic review. Neurology 2002;58:1327–1332.

7. Struck, AF, Ustun, B, Ruiz, AR, Lee, JW, LaRoche, SM, Hirsch, LJ, et al. Association of an electroen-cephalography-based risk score with seizure probability in hospitalized patients. JAMA Neurol 2017; 74:1419–1424.

8. Tatum, WO, Olga, S, Ochoa, JG, Munger Clary, H, Cheek, J, Drislane, F, et al. American Clinical Neurophysiology Society Guideline 7: Guidelines for EEG reporting. J Clin Neurophysiol 2016; 33:328–332.

Index

Note: Locators in *italics* represent figures and **bold** indicate tables in the text.